Unmentionable Madness

DISABILITY HISTORIES

Series editors: Stephanie Hunt-Kennedy, Kim E. Nielsen, and Michael Rembis

Disability Histories seeks scholarship that explores the lived experiences of individuals and groups from a broad range of societies, cultures, time periods, and geographic locations, who either identified as disabled or were considered by the dominant culture to be disabled.

We conceive of disability and disabled experiences broadly and seek to include scholarship that spans a range of embodiments, including the emerging field of mad studies. We are especially interested in scholarship that not only employs innovative approaches to using disability—in constant interaction with systems of race, class, gender, and sexuality—as an analytical tool to deepen our understanding of larger power relations, ideologies, and institutions, but also engages in meaningful dialogue with other subdisciplines within history, such as legal and political histories, social histories, histories of technology, science, and medicine, histories of the body and sexuality, and histories of the development of capitalism and imperialism. We welcome submissions from a variety of geopolitical locations, especially those that situate disability history outside European and North American contexts, including regions or nations that would become identified as the "Global South." We are interested in scholarship that moves beyond traditional disability frameworks and offers methodologies and approaches to disability history that are rooted in decolonial, transnational, and transimperial perspectives.

For a list of books in the series, please see our website at www.press.uillinois.edu.

UNMENTIONABLE MADNESS

Gender, Disability, and Shame in the Malaria Treatment of Neurosyphilis

CHRISTIN L. HANCOCK

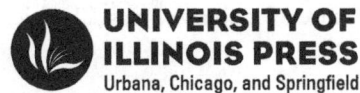

© 2025 by the Board of Trustees
of the University of Illinois
All rights reserved
1 2 3 4 5 C P 5 4 3 2 1
♾ This book is printed on acid-free paper.

Library of Congress Cataloging-in-Publication Data

Names: Hancock, Christin Lee, 1974– author.
Title: Unmentionable madness : gender, disability, and shame in the malaria treatment of neurosyphilis / Christin L. Hancock.
Description: Urbana : University of Illinois Press, [2025] | Series: Disability histories | Includes bibliographical references and index.
Identifiers: LCCN 2024024207 (print) | LCCN 2024024208 (ebook) | ISBN 9780252046148 (cloth) | ISBN 9780252088223 (paperback) | ISBN 9780252047404 (ebook)
Subjects: LCSH: People with disabilities—Social conditions. | Human experimentation in medicine. | People with disabilities—Abuse of. | Discrimination against people with disabilities. | Neurosyphilis—Treatment.
Classification: LCC HV1552 .H36 2025 (print) | LCC HV1552 (ebook) | DDC 362.4—dc23/eng/20240918
LC record available at https://lccn.loc.gov/2024024207
LC ebook record available at https://lccn.loc.gov/2024024208

To Mabel and all the unnamed women and men who died at Central State Hospital.

And to Tom, Liam, Silé, and Micah, with all my love.

Contents

Acknowledgments   ix

Introduction: Mabel Smith, Ancestral Disability, and Shame   1

1 Mabel Smith   17

2 Dr. Walter L. Bruetsch   37

3 Supplying the Research: Patient Experiences at CSH   59

4 Race, Gender, and Neurosyphilis   83

5 Dying from Neurosyphilis and the Silencing of Disability   103

Conclusion: Revisiting Mabel, Dismantling Shame   119

Notes   125

Bibliography   153

Index   165

Acknowledgments

Having begun this project nearly eight years ago, I have acquired many debts of gratitude. To begin, thanks to my sister Lorie Kefeitz. Without her curiosity and tenacity in first requesting Mabel's medical file more than two decades ago, this book would not exist. I am thankful for our shared history and friendship. Lorie generously read every word of the manuscript, and for that I am also grateful.

Thanks to my mom, Mary, and her many siblings—my aunts and uncles—who expressed their interest in my pursuit of Mabel's story. During one of my research visits, many of them sat in the backyard of my Aunt Kay's house and talked with me about what they knew, and mostly did not know, about Mabel. Thanks to my dad, Jeff, who drove me to Illinois to visit my first archive for my sixth grade History Day project. Thanks to my sister Stacie for visits during my research trips. My grandparents Rosemary and Tom died many years ago, but I am ever grateful to them for creating a welcoming home for me and my siblings, cousins, and friends. As a child I spent numerous Sunday afternoons spinning stories for my younger cousins, who sat stacked up on a narrow staircase that spilled into the dining room, eagerly listening to tales mostly plucked from my imagination. Now, here's a real story.

Institutional support is critical to any years-long historical research project such as this. Thanks to the University of Portland for providing this support in the form of sabbatical leaves, which made possible the time to conduct research and writing, and Butine Grants, which supported research trips and multiple academic conference presentations. Several colleagues at the University of Portland read and offered feedback on early versions of this work. Thanks so much to Laurie McClary, Allie Stewart, Terry Favero, and Cara Hersh for your thoughtful engagement. Thanks also to my University of Portland writing group, including Molly Hiro, Rachel Wheeler, Brandy Daniels, Matthew Warshawsky, Kristin Sweeney, Alexa Dare, Anne Santiago, and Neil Oculi. During the pandemic this group kept me engaged and on track. Additional University of Portland colleagues have provided meaningful support along the way, including my colleagues in the Gender, Women, and Sexuality Studies program and the Department of History. Thanks, too, to Karen Eifler, Shaz Vijlee, and Jeff Meiser. And thanks to my undergraduate history majors who have eagerly engaged the histories of "madness," disability, and gender over the past several years, helping me sharpen my own thinking in the process.

Molly Hiro, Amy Donogue, Alice Gates, and Erin Kelley have provided steady friendship across the years that includes support of this project and all the little milestones along the way. Karen Inouye's friendship and sense of humor always lift my spirits. Cecilia Tsu read early versions of this work and has regularly encouraged me to keep going. Valerie Francisco-Menchavez reminded me early on that this is a story that needs to be told. Thanks to Joel Frieburger for cajoling me into attending a writing conference with him. Kimberly Jensen and Febe Pamonag have become treasured collaborators and friends throughout the years of this work. Kim became my first enthusiastic supporter when I tentatively shared the idea for this book with her in the basement of the Oregon Historical Society. She envisioned this book as real and meaningful even before I was able to believe it myself. Febe and I met on a conference panel five years ago, and we have been happily collaborating ever since. Thanks to them both for years of shared intellectual passion, academic presentations, and friendship.

At the University of Notre Dame, Gail Bederman inspired me through her teaching of women's and gender history, and in the process, she modeled a career as a historian for this uncertain undergraduate. At Brown University Mari Jo Buhle taught me everything about historical research and writing; my work as a historian is undoubtedly better thanks to her high standards and rigorous expectations. For that, as well as her enthusiasm about this project, I am ever grateful.

Archivists and librarians play an essential role in any historical research work, and this book is no exception. I am immensely grateful to Claire Alderfer, director of the Indiana State Archives, for her years of tireless efforts in locating and facilitating access to critical sources. I met Claire on my very first research trip to Indiana, and I am indebted to her for ongoing support of my research over the past eight years as well as her compassion and care in preserving the state of Indiana's important historical records. Thanks to Claire and the other members of the Indiana Archives and Records Administration Privacy Committee for supporting research that helps destigmatize mental illness and for protecting privacy in the process. Thanks to Sarah Halter of the Indiana Medical History Museum for multiple helpful communications (in person and via email), and to David Bartolowits at St. John the Evangelist Catholic Church, who provided helpful assistance with church records. And many thanks to the librarians and student workers at my own campus library who have assisted over the years with my never-ending requests for more interlibrary loans.

I am indebted to the many incredible scholars who have read this work and generously shared their expertise and wisdom to improve it. Thanks to Deirdre Cooper Owens, who provided insightful feedback on a very early conference presentation, pointing me to the important work of Barbara Fields and Karen Fields. Thanks to Geoffrey Reaume and Erika Dyck, who, in their roles as readers for the press, provided substantive and astute feedback on the book proposal and some early chapters. Several additional anonymous readers provided excellent and helpful suggestions both in the early and later stages. The book is undoubtedly better than it would have been thanks to the insights of all these scholars. Disability Histories series editors Stephanie Hunt-Kennedy, Kim E. Nielsen, and Michael Rembis have been amazing. They have engaged generously with the entire manuscript, providing perceptive feedback and specific suggestions that helped me clarify my arguments and correct my errors at multiple points throughout the process. Their collective deep commitment to the field of disability studies, and their care and thoughtfulness in guiding my work, has meant everything. Alison Syring at the University of Illinois Press is a fantastic reader, and she has been incredibly helpful in ushering this book into being. Thanks, too, to Jessica Hinds-Bond for meticulous copyediting, and to Leigh Ann Cowan and everyone else at the press for the behind-the-scenes production work that has made the book a reality.

Liam, Silé, and Micah Rinehart have grown up alongside this book, with the younger two sometimes accompanying me on research trips to Indianapolis. These three wonderful humans are bright lights in the world, and I'm so lucky and thankful to be their mother. And, finally, tremendous thanks to Tom Rinehart: the very best husband and friend, a true partner in all things, fantastic father to our children, provider of music and beauty, witty and smart conversationalist, the person with whom I always want to discuss everything, reader of every chapter of this book many times over. I am eternally grateful that I get to live this life with Tom.

Unmentionable Madness

Introduction
Mabel Smith, Ancestral Disability, and Shame

On October 18, 1930, Arthur Smith drove his young wife, Mabel, up the long, paved drive of the Central State Hospital for the Insane (CSH) in Indianapolis, Indiana. On wide acreage several miles south of the downtown core, CSH's main building towered over the acres of dewy autumn grass surrounding it. Passing through the main gate, twenty-eight-year-old Mabel stared blankly out the car window, eyes crossed. With no history of insanity, Mabel had suddenly lost her sense of reasoning, becoming "confused, incoherent," and "maniacal."[1] She had been first taken to City Hospital, but her physical and mental condition deteriorated; doctors decided to transfer Mabel, like so many other "paretics" before her, to CSH for care of her advanced mental troubles.[2] Upon her admission, Mabel's Wassermann test confirmed what the physician on duty already suspected: Mabel suffered from neurosyphilis, a late-stage disease process of syphilis that affects the nervous system and induces insanity. In January 1931 physicians at CSH injected Mabel with malaria in an effort to cure her insanity. Six weeks later she was dead.[3]

In the 1920s and 1930s untreated syphilis infection accounted for the insanity of as much as 20 percent of patients in US public asylums; for most it was a death sentence.[4] And yet despite its dangerous prevalence, the American public struggled to talk about both sexuality and the consequences of venereal disease, making prevention especially difficult. Early regular treatment of syphilis, which by the first decade of the twentieth century involved an arsenical compound called Salvarsan, could potentially halt the disease progression; yet many Americans, embarrassed—even shamed—by the stigma associated with syphilis, failed to be diagnosed or treated.[5] Women in particular bore the brunt of shame associated with sexually transmitted infections, as their illnesses revealed their apparent promiscuity.[6] Illness, disability, and institutionalization imprinted these sexual transgressions on women's physical bodies, highlighting their moral delinquencies for an attentive public.

Desperate for a cure for what was believed to be a public health scourge, a small group of American psychiatrists in the 1920s rallied around the promising research of Austrian physician Julius Wagner-Jauregg, who proposed inoculating paretic patients—those suffering from neurosyphilis—with malaria. Over the course of the next two decades, psychiatrists at state mental hospitals around the nation embarked on sustained programs of malaria therapy treatment, with CSH in Indianapolis serving as a leader among them. After being injected with malaria, women and men suffered repeated, painful, high fever spikes, often over the course of several weeks. Physicians, who focused on "cure," hoped the malaria infection would end the debilitating impairments caused by neurosyphilis infection.[7] Although researchers claimed success with "fever therapy," recording a cure rate of between 25 and 30 percent, its actual efficacy remains largely uncertain.[8] And yet for a short but important time in the 1920s and 1930s malaria therapy was the treatment of choice for "general paralysis of the insane."[9] Viewing malaria therapy as a potential magic bullet, researchers typically overlooked the pain, exhaustion, debility, and danger associated with the treatment itself, largely erasing disabled women and men's experiences of this "cure."[10]

Using a feminist disability studies framework, this book argues that the popular but ethically ambiguous medical research project known as malaria therapy—an experimental treatment conducted on institutionalized patients at CSH for more than two decades—depended on the increasingly disabled minds and bodies of those incarcerated to establish its "success." As one scholar explains, feminist disability studies, which foregrounds embodied experiences, explores the ways diverse physical bodies have interacted with "their social and material environments."[11] I employ this approach by highlighting women's embodied experiences of illness and severe impairments in a historical context that demanded gender conformity and "normalcy."[12] The malaria treatment both reflected and perpetuated social biases about poverty, gender, race, and disability, as well as an overarching desire to protect the public from people who were perceived as abnormal and unworthy of community life. Unfolding during a period of time when eugenic theory gained prominence in American medicine, guiding medical researchers' beliefs about all the aforementioned identities, malaria therapy ultimately embraced the notion that the community benefited from the experimental medical treatment of persons deemed "unfit," regardless of the individual physical and emotional costs of that treatment.[13] As a result, inequalities of power both created and sustained this ethically questionable biomedical treatment and research at CSH, even as the daily practices and theoretical conclusions of the research project itself solidified socially constructed meanings of gender, race, and (dis)ability.

Mabel Smith's story, shocking though it may sound, was not particularly unique, given the significant numbers of insane asylum patients who suffered from somatic illness. But her story is one that has not often been told, both because of the historical challenges involved in recovering voices of the institutionalized and because of the languishing of such stories in family shame and secrecy. As scholars of affect and emotion have noted, shame is both an individual emotional experience and a construct of community and social relationships.[14] Indeed, central to the individual's experience of shame is the presence of an audience that judges.[15] As a historical object, shame sheds light not only on individual experiences of pain, but also on the ways that communities construct meanings about social values and expectations that ultimately shape identity. Shame—as differentiated from guilt—tends to focus on the core self rather than a behavior or misdeed that can be corrected.[16] Historian Peter N. Stearns notes that as a result of this focus on the self, shame "creates greater pain and intensity than guilt," leading to urgent attempts at "denying" and "forgetting."[17] Thus it is perhaps not surprising that shame and silence go hand in hand. The shame associated with sexual transgression, madness, and institutionalization has, as a rather common consequence of the emotion itself, frequently resulted in family erasure through concerted efforts to deny or forget intensely painful experiences.

I first learned about Mabel Smith as an adolescent, eavesdropping on the kitchen table conversation of my mother, her sisters, and my grandmother, none of whom seemed entirely certain what had happened to her. My great-aunt had died in the state mental hospital, and in the 1980s this was not something that anyone felt was very appropriate to talk about, particularly within earshot of her brother, my grandfather. Mabel's shame during her lifetime had morphed into a family shame, carried by her parents and siblings into their future lives, from which a pervasive silence emanated. The whispered kitchen talk from my youth revealed little of substance about Mabel's life or death. In the late 1990s, prompted by her growing interest in psychology and mental health, my sister, Lorie Keifetz, requested Mabel's medical file from the Indiana State Archives, which is how we discovered her syphilis diagnosis and her treatment with malaria therapy. This information stuck with me throughout graduate school and the early years of my career as an academic historian, despite my feeling as though I did not have time to pursue it. Nearly eight years ago, during my first sabbatical, my ongoing curiosity about the larger historical context of Mabel's diagnosis and treatment prompted me to begin tracking down both the details of her story and the larger history surrounding her. Although in the 1920s and 1930s medical reports documenting malaria therapy highlighted the promising number of people who recovered from neurosyphilis, I wondered about the overwhelming majority—those like Mabel—who had died either despite or because of the treatment. I began to conduct research into the fuller context of this unknown aunt's life and death alongside the historical narrative of the experimental malaria treatment.

In reconstructing my Aunt Mabel's story, I am in part doing the "repair" work that Jennifer Natalya Fink calls "re-lineating," seeking out and claiming my disabled ancestor who was silenced in both life and death, and ultimately erased from my kinship story. For Fink, re-creating family lineages to include disabled ancestors who have previously been de-lineated through shame and silence restores a more holistic picture of kinship even as it challenges ableism and promotes healing by making disability normative in our family stories.[18] In the process of re-lineating, I am also making a particular claim that shame and silence surrounding family disability—though perhaps universally practiced in "all our families"—are historically and culturally specific, such that these common practices of erasure look and function differently in varied contexts.[19] Specific historical moments combined with variables of race, socioeconomic class, religion, gendered expectations, and region all work together to shape the particular experience of shame and silence. For instance, for me, someone who grew up in the 1970s and 1980s within a large extended white working- to middle-class Catholic family, disability at birth and the disability that accompanies aging were both more or less accepted as normative parts of life.[20] By contrast, *acquired disability* resulted in shame and the persistent secrecy that accompanied it. Acquired disabilities—in this case, mental and emotional anguish brought about by transgressive sexuality—suggested "defective" behavior that was treated as such.[21] Thus, in telling Mabel's particular story of acquired disability, I am normalizing her sexual behavior as well as her experience of mental and physical debility and institutionalization, all of which were considered aberrant and shameful during her life as well as after her death. In the process I am, as Fink says, "sew[ing]" her "back into the patchwork quilt of our family's story."[22] In making Mabel and her disability both visible and familiar, I hope that I am also reducing shame. After all, when we stop trying to deny or forget, and allow ourselves to look clearly at the past, things that appeared "strange" or "unfamiliar" become less so.[23]

In addition to re-lineating, in telling Mabel's story I am also stitching together a history of disability in conversation with a sociomedical history about a largely overlooked experimental medical treatment. Although relatively few historians have written specifically about malaria therapy, my research is indebted to a small group of scholars who have previously engaged the topic. Joel Braslow's study of a Southern California mental institution that began its malaria treatment several years after CSH argues that malaria therapy gave physicians a sense of hope that positively shifted their perceptions of their patients. Although my conclusions about malaria therapy at CSH differ from Braslow's, his work nonetheless provides an invaluable model for employing an institutional history as a case study, even as it also points to the important social relationship between patient and healer.[24] Several other historians have explored additional aspects of malaria therapy history that have been instrumental to my thinking. These scholars include Margaret Humphreys, who traces the history of the malariologist Mark Boyd's work with syphilis patients in Florida; Matthew Gambino, who looks at the malaria therapy experiment at Saint Elizabeths Hospital in Washington, DC; and Susan M. Reverby, who includes a chapter on Dr. Eugene H. Dibble Jr. and malaria treatment at the Veterans Hospital in Tuskegee, Alabama, in her history of the infamous Tuskegee study, which withheld syphilis treatment from Black men.[25] My research builds on the work of each of these important scholars and yet also establishes its own unique contribution in terms of its arguments and structure, as well as its new/unexamined evidence as found in the case study of CSH. Specifically, by centering patient experiences, my research prioritizes questions about shame, disability, pain, and the ways medical treatments construct "normalcy."

The grueling malaria treatment, which sought to return mentally and physically disabled women and men to the status of "normal," productive, and noninstitutionalized, was neither easy to endure nor necessarily good for the majority of those who received it. Although medical researchers and asylum leaders believed in the "goodness" of their work, they nonetheless embarked on medical experimentation on medically incarcerated people whom they believed to be "abnormal." As such, telling Mabel's story along with the stories of hundreds of others who—like her—ultimately succumbed to neurosyphilis despite medical treatment that was meant to cure, provides a blueprint for writing medical history that not only engages with but centers disability history in the storytelling.[26]

In constructing this history, this book prioritizes the voices of women (and men) who died at CSH during their medical incarceration. Although voices of institutionalized women can be particularly challenging to uncover, women and gender historians as well as "mad studies" scholars and disability historians have done a remarkable job piecing together these experiences.[27] Giving voice to some of the hundreds of patients who suffered from neurosyphilis, found themselves institutionalized and inoculated with malaria, and ultimately died, this book foregrounds their experiences and their involuntary roles in medical experimentation through a careful examination of institutional and archival records (also known as "authoritative sources"), in combination with less frequently utilized genealogical history and material culture sources.[28] Although many of my sources represent official documents created by superintendents, psychiatrists, and medical researchers, I approach these sources critically, reading them for subtle clues that reveal patients' perspectives and experiences.[29] Centering feminist disability history helps to decenter medical history as the one authoritative account of the history of disease and illness.

Over the past several years I have pored over patient files, research notes, medical journals, newspaper articles, birth and death certificates, and church and hospital records in an effort to understand the ways Mabel and patients like her experienced their disabilities and death in the context of the malaria therapy treatment. In addition to conducting archival research, I spent many weeks in Indianapolis, walking in and around the physical spaces that Mabel Smith inhabited, seeking to connect my archival research to my own physical experience of space and place.[30] As part of this research process, I visited the Indiana Medical History Museum, housed in the old pathology building on the campus of the former CSH, where much of the original malaria therapy research was conducted. Driving onto the grounds of the state asylum where Mabel died, walking around and into the pathology building where Dr. Bruetsch dissected disabled bodies, I sensed the weightiness of the silence surrounding my great-aunt's life and death. I have spent time driving around the neighborhood where Mabel lived; many of the street addresses no longer correspond to houses, freeways and urban development cutting into the spaces that bordered Mabel's life. I have walked downtown Indianapolis, stopping in at St. John's Catholic parish to examine sacramental record books, and at the Indiana State Department of Health Vital Records office to request copies of death certificates. And I have visited the cemetery where Mabel is buried, locating her small overgrown headstone, which lies unassuming near a small tree. I should also add that throughout these journeys, I have been consistently greeted with incredibly kind, generous, and interested research help from archivists and museum directors, as well as city, parish, and funeral home employees. This visitation work has contributed to the care I have tried to bring to my reading of the sources.[31]

Dr. Walter Bruetsch, Madness, and Malaria Therapy at Central State Hospital

My research into malaria therapy led me to multiple archives in Indianapolis, where I first encountered Dr. Walter L. Bruetsch in addition to hundreds of his patients. Although a state-run insane asylum in Indiana may seem an unlikely setting for experimental treatments, CSH played a leading role in the nation's malaria therapy treatment of syphilis, becoming one of the first institutions to begin and sustain a multiyear malaria therapy research practice.[32] In large part due to the work of German-born pathologist and lead researcher Dr. Bruetsch, CSH became a major center for biomedical research. Trained by Wagner-Jauregg himself, Dr. Bruetsch committed decades of his life's work to the study of malaria-treated neurosyphilis, and the patients at CSH became the research material that made his work possible.

Because there is no centralized database of malaria-treated patients in the Indiana State Archives, only those patients whom the experiment failed are traceable. Given this reality, I worked backward through autopsy records and obituaries to collect a partial list of patients who died from neurosyphilis at CSH from 1925 to 1945. Working through these records alongside the hospital's annual reports and other official documents importantly interrupts a long-standing historical silence.[33] As it turns out, Dr. Bruetsch's research project entirely depended on the patients who died, even if they, in turn, did not end up reaping the rewards promised by his "beneficence."[34] The stigma and shame that surrounded Mabel and women like her in life clung to her even in death, such that her story has remained absent not only from personal family histories and memories, but also from a wider historical discussion of the experimental medical treatment. Shame reverberated throughout Mabel's experience and throughout the stories of loss and death that unfold here.

Perhaps because women accounted for a minority of syphilis patients around the nation, even those histories that do explore the malaria therapy treatment have tended to focus more broadly on male patients, overlooking both women's stories and any particularly gendered aspects of this history. This lack of attention erases women's experiences. It also leaves intact the (erroneous) gendered presumption that men suffered from madness caused by somatic illness and women did not.[35] As such it further perpetuates the notion that women have not experienced the painful realities of mental and physical impairment caused by madness. And yet as the history of the malaria treatment demonstrates, women did indeed experience neurosyphilis-induced madness, which left them paralyzed, hallucinating, isolated, lonely, scared, and ultimately dying.

The feminist disability studies approach employed here resituates women in this narrative of malaria therapy treatment. Despite the clear historical existence of women's neurological impairment, women's material experiences of madness have often been overlooked in favor of what Elizabeth J. Donaldson calls "the figure of the madwoman as feminist rebel."[36] As Donaldson demonstrates, feminist theory's emphasis on the ways that psychiatry unfairly pathologized women—especially women who broke gender barriers—though important, has perhaps unintentionally limited scholarly exploration of women's bodily experiences of mental impairment. By contrast, Donaldson calls for a feminist disability studies approach to the history of madness, one that "demands closer attention to physical bodies and to the theories of embodiment."[37] Taking up this call, my historical study of the malaria therapy experience draws on feminist disability studies, placing women's bodies and embodied experiences of madness at the center of the study.[38] Such historical positioning places my work in what Michael Rembis calls the "liminal space between a medicalized or biologized notion of madness and a more social or relational understanding of what it means to live a 'mad' existence."[39] Through highlighting these individual patient stories alongside the institutional history of CSH's malaria therapy treatment, I hope to create a fuller picture of how (dis)ability was constructed along gendered lines during the interwar era. In this way, the book uncovers the story of an illness and its treatment by centering the stories of those people who suffered from that illness.[40]

This history also importantly engages the larger history of psychiatric institutionalization and what several scholars have referred to as the "carceral state" in the first half of the twentieth-century United States.[41] In the early twentieth century, Progressive Era reformers as well as medical activists and others in the "helping professions" sought to protect the public from the perceived dangers presented by the mad and degenerate.[42] As part of this realm of "help," the incarceration of mad people in asylums established and solidified a professional class of medical providers whose professional careers depended on continued incarceration of mad people. Institutionalized against their will, women and men suffering from neurosyphilis found themselves caught in a cycle of "help" that identified them as disabled, in need of social isolation, supervision, and medical care. And yet for the majority of those treated with malaria therapy, the medical care did little to improve their situations. By contrast, the malaria treatment and research did much to burnish the modern medical credentials of CSH and the medical men who led it. At CSH, the bodies of women and men suffering severe impairment became the locus of experimental learning that helped solidify the professional reputation of both the institution and its leaders.[43]

Situating this story within the context of disability history provides the important and generative opportunity to question the ways that ableism has shaped medical research and the experience of shame. In many ways Dr. Bruetsch was then and is still heralded a hero. At the Indiana Medical History Museum, a large painting of a serious, thoughtful Bruetsch hangs in the reception room greeting visitors. Living as he did in an apartment on the hospital grounds, Bruetsch worked all hours of the day with single-minded focus. Although social and medical reformers at the time as well as perhaps some medical historians today laud(ed) Bruetsch's all-consuming desire to find a cure for the dreaded paresis, he nonetheless played a complicated role in the lives of his patients. As the medical authority in charge of research, Dr. Bruetsch shaped their experiences of institutionalization and medical incarceration. Because the purpose of this history is to question rather than condemn, centering the story on Mabel's (and others') experience of disability allows us to move beyond conversations about medical intentions and efficacy, opening up space for critical inquiry of medical practices and ideas that are sometimes perceived to be beyond reproach.[44] Women and men who found themselves at CSH rarely arrived there voluntarily. As such, even when and where they existed, physicians' good intentions did not mitigate patients' experiences of fear, pain, violence, and shame.

Regardless of the intentions of Progressive Era medical men, patients at CSH experienced institutionalization and malaria treatment as carceral in shape and structure.[45] Dr. Bruetsch oversaw the last days of life for many who died from neurosyphilis and malaria therapy. As the lead pathologist, he took apart many of their bodies in the wake of their deaths. It was Bruetsch's hands that held their syphilitic brains and hearts outside of their bodies, carefully weighing and cutting and examining. In a historical moment that preceded the evolution of official laws regarding informed consent and patient rights, Bruetsch's relationship to his patients both before and after their deaths seems particularly important to understanding medical experimentation within the context of institutionalization and the social and cultural values surrounding ability and disability that are so deeply embedded within that story. Anchoring this history in the experiences of disabled women and men helps us reshift focus from judgments about intentions and efficacy to interrogations about the experience of shame, pain, and illness and about the way that concepts such as cure, success, and normalcy get shaped and defined.

Historical Context: Eugenics, Madness, and Neurosyphilis

The sexually transmitted infection known as syphilis has a long and global history, one that has been widely documented by social historians.⁴⁶ Left untreated, syphilis could spread to the brain, resulting in neurosyphilis, which caused physical paralysis, loss of speech and memory, severe dementia, hallucinations, emotional disturbances, and eventually death. The horror of the potential progression of the disease, combined with the high rates of syphilitic infection, prompted Progressive Era public health reformers, medical doctors, and psychiatrists to urgently campaign against the disease, despite the social taboos breached by such public conversation about sex and venereal disease. Medical breakthroughs, which aided in diagnosis and treatment of early-stage syphilis in the early years of the twentieth century, contributed to this concerted public push toward prevention.⁴⁷ These advances also provided a biological basis for the cause of mental impairment, ultimately displacing nineteenth-century beliefs in immorality as a primary cause. New medical discoveries about syphilis fit neatly within the broader transitions in psychiatric perceptions about insanity.⁴⁸

An expanding medical embrace of eugenics accompanied and shaped this shift in psychiatric perceptions about the causes of madness. It was within this context of the growing popularity of eugenic thinking, which sought to protect the public against those deemed "unfit," that Progressive Era reformers urgently sought a solution to the public health crisis posed by untreated syphilis infection. Thus, although reformers, psychiatrists, and leaders of state mental institutions appeared in some ways to be operating on the cutting edge of progressive reform, their campaigns often overlapped with eugenic rhetoric and practices that reinforced biased assumptions about ability and disability. Although World War I had provided the context for the first federally funded public health discourse about venereal disease, in the aftermath of the war, that relative openness—in addition to the funding—dried up. During the 1920s, American public attitudes returned to the prewar realm of social taboo, shame, and stigma.⁴⁹ At the national level, the 1936 elevation of Dr. Thomas Parran to the position of US surgeon general helped revitalize the wartime commitment to science in public health, as Parran fought to bring venereal disease education back into the national discourse in his crusade against syphilis. In the process, he relied on the rhetoric of eugenics to help shape and validate the work.⁵⁰ It was also about this time, in 1932, that the US Public Health Service began its infamous experiment at Tuskegee, in which treatment was withheld from Black men suffering from syphilis.⁵¹

Reflections of popular eugenics played out among the reforming efforts of public health professionals at the local level, and perhaps nowhere was this more evident than in the state of Indiana. As with the national context, the local context included desperate efforts to confront an urgent public health crisis. These efforts in the name of public health contributed to the state's early and continued political embrace of eugenics.[52] Superintendent of CSH, Dr. Max Bahr, became one of those public health reformers whose desire to curb a public health scourge led to the support of state policies steeped in eugenic thinking. In a 1917 speech delivered before the Indiana Health Conference and Health Officers School, Dr. Bahr—then clinical psychiatrist at CSH—noted that "paresis is a particularly fatal disease, and no treatment as yet has been found to cure it." Statistics, he argued, did not capture the full story, as social stigma motivated many families to bring their "paretics" home from mental institutions in order to hide the true cause of their impending deaths. Families hoped to spare their fatally ill loved one from being labeled with "such a dreaded disease, for," as Bahr noted, "the laity are quite well informed of the fact that paresis means syphilis."[53] For Bahr, both the devastation and the family shame wrought by syphilis represented a public health emergency for which communities were responsible. As such, Bahr argued in favor of a public health registry of syphilitic patients that would prohibit them from obtaining marriage licenses until after they received medical clearance. Some twenty years later, Bahr's efforts found success when, in 1940, Indiana joined eighteen other states in passing a marriage blood test law, which required both marriage license applicants to be tested for syphilis.[54] Such "eugenics marriage laws" were born out of public health goals that sought to prohibit the procreation of those deemed unfit.[55] Although Indiana eventually, in 1987, repealed this blood test requirement, its passage represented the culmination of decades of public health activism aimed at tackling the problems posed by syphilis.[56] Seeking to avoid not only the impairment but also the shame caused by neurosyphilis, Indiana public health leaders in tandem with state institutions like CSH leaned into the eugenic thinking that reverberated throughout their reforming efforts.

This book tracks the history of the experimental malaria therapy treatment of syphilis-induced madness through the life stories of patient and researcher. Lining up Mabel Smith and her experience of disability alongside Dr. Walter Bruetsch's work at CSH allows for multiple avenues of exploration of a story that at its heart engages issues of power and inequality, shame and silence. Beyond re-lineating Mabel within my own family lineage, restoring Mabel's and other patients' voices alongside the better-known voice of the lead pathologist of CSH, who became a world-renowned medical researcher, helps rebalance the power between these unequally situated historical actors. Indeed, it is unlikely that Mabel could have ever expected to be remembered in a book, and perhaps it is equally unlikely that Dr. Bruetsch would have anticipated his patients being given such a platform from which to speak about the complicated story of their involuntary interactions over madness, syphilis, and malaria. The book, then, in its format, seeks to rebalance power even as it offers up a critique of the historical inequities of power evident in the unequal relationships between medical providers and those experiencing disability caused by neurosyphilis. The book opens with the story of Mabel's life, followed by the story of Dr. Bruetsch at CSH. From there, the book zooms out from these microhistories to explore larger themes based on hundreds of patient experiences of pain, illness, and institutionalization; the ways that medical treatment, observation, and experimentation resulted in constructions of race, gender, and "normalcy"; and, finally, patient deaths and the role of autopsy in the continued medical research project. Throughout these thematic explorations, Mabel Smith's life and death serve as touch points, revealing the historical particularities of shame and madness in her story.

Chapter 1, which introduces Mabel Dalton Smith, argues that sexual deviance and neurosyphilis doubly stigmatized young women, rendering them "abnormal" and in need of sequestering from the "healthy" community. The chapter details Mabel's biography, tracing the cultural and social change that occurred during her lifetime as well as illuminating the social, political, religious, and economic world of the south side of Indianapolis in the period of 1900–1930. Beginning as it does with the biography of a woman who suffered illness and death, this chapter importantly establishes neurosyphilis and the malaria therapy as disability history. Chapter 2 introduces Dr. Walter Bruetsch and his work at CSH, arguing that he was hired in the role of pathologist with the specific intention of creating a research program designed to improve the prestige of CSH. The urgent desire to find cures for insanity in the 1920s, which prompted the usage of increasingly radical experimental therapies, underscores my own claim that Dr. Bruetsch had a vested professional interest in bringing malaria therapy to Indianapolis.⁵⁷ Chapter 3 examines the full context of the malaria treatment of syphilis and its impact on individual patients. Analysis of patients' stories and their experiences forms the backbone of this chapter, which argues that the inequalities between the institution and people experiencing disability created the context for a steady stream of research participants who had little choice about their health or medical future. Chapter 4 explores these power inequalities as they relate to race and gender in more detail. This chapter argues that the racialized findings of Dr. Bruetsch both reflected and contributed to the larger national and international medical discourse that engaged eugenic thinking and medical racism. This chapter also argues that definitions of "success" were predicated on gendered ideas about ability and productive labor, all of which further reflected the eugenic thinking that predominated at the time. Finally, chapter 5 examines the role of death and autopsy in malaria therapy research, arguing that marginalized patients who supplied the research material for this experimental treatment in life, continued to do so in and after death.

Throughout this work, I have regularly reflected on my own ethical responsibilities as a researcher and as a (currently) nondisabled historian of disability. I have worked very hard to treat the lives, health, and death stories of individuals who died while institutionalized with great care and respect.⁵⁸ Struggling to determine how I might intervene in the larger historical narrative of medical experimentation without replicating the ethical ambiguities that my study critiques, I have followed the lead of historians of disability and madness who have argued for the importance of centering the stories of those experiencing madness while also protecting individual privacy.⁵⁹ As Mabel's grand-niece, I have decided to tell her story in its entirety, or at least in the entirety that I have been able to piece together. Committed as I am to destigmatizing both mental disability and the perceived sexual transgressions of women, I am grateful to be able to breathe life into Mabel's story, returning her not only to my family lineage, but to a larger historical discussion of the interconnections of sexuality and disability. In the process, I hope the telling of her story eases the shame she and her immediate family members experienced through her illness and death. And, although Mabel may have been surprised to find herself the subject of a book, I very much hope (and like to think) that she would be pleased by it. In order to protect the privacy and personal health information of all other women and men who lived and died as patients at CSH, I have anonymized patient files and information gathered from them. In a few cases, I have created pseudonyms, and in these instances, I have included an endnote indicating as much. In all cases I am grateful for the opportunity that I have had to learn from these embodied experiences of mental impairment, and I hope that I have done justice to the stories of women and men who died at CSH. This work is dedicated to them.

CHAPTER 1

Mabel Smith

On October 18, 1930, a Central State Hospital (CSH) physician named Dr. Tidwell conducted an intake with a young emaciated white woman who had been transferred that day from City Hospital, the downtown Indianapolis hospital that served the city's poor. As he recorded case number 16086, Dr. Tidwell noted that Mabel Smith was a "housewife... 28 years of age, very thin and nervous." Mabel stood five feet six and a half inches tall and weighed barely 108 pounds. She had dark hair and "numerous freckles" scattered about the otherwise clear complexion of her pale face. Describing her condition, Dr. Tidwell observed that Mabel arrived with a staggering gait, "degeneracy of face and head," crossed eyes and sluggish pupils, and a speech defect, and behaved in a "silly, maniacal" manner, with a "complete loss of reasoning and judgment."[1] Although Mabel denied having either syphilis or gonorrhea, her positive Wassermann test and her spinal fluid stated otherwise. Dr. Tidwell recorded her diagnosis: "general paralysis of the insane." Mabel Smith suffered from neurosyphilis, the physically and mentally devastating tertiary stage of syphilis, a fatal condition that accounted for 20 percent of patients' admissions at state institutions nationwide.

Upon patients' arrival at CSH, doctors evaluated and treated them in the medical ward, also called the "admission unit," for six months in the hopes that treatment would offer a cure—or, in the absence of a cure, at least what CSH superintendent Max Bahr referred to as a "trial furlough" return to home. At the end of that initial admission period, those patients who failed to improve enough to be discharged were transferred to longer-term regular wards.[2] These patients became lifelong occupants of the hospital, their hopes for recovery or release diminishing with each passing year. After her arrival at CSH that October day, Mabel never made it out of the admission unit. As the year came to an end, and fall turned into winter, the medical team in charge of Mabel's case determined that she should receive CSH's malaria therapy treatment, and so on January 3, 1931, medical staff at CSH inoculated Mabel with malaria. From the third of January through the twenty-first, Mabel lay in the medical ward, where she experienced repeated malarial fever spikes.[3] Presumably doctors then administered quinine to halt the malaria infection, though this is not recorded in her patient file. If Mabel's husband, Arthur Smith, had hoped to bring his young wife home to their residence at 5230 West McCarty Street, those hopes were dashed when Mabel succumbed to general paralysis of the insane on February 27, 1931.[4]

Toward the end of her short life Mabel's acquired disability caused severe mental and physical impairment that ultimately led to her institutionalized death. Although she entered CSH as a seemingly properly married woman, Mabel's predisability life harbored shameful secrets that she and her husband had tried to bury. Nearly a decade prior, Mabel had engaged in a sexual relationship with a young boyfriend that resulted in both a pregnancy and a hastily arranged first marriage. At a historical moment when single working-class women were increasingly exploring their sexuality even as any public evidence of that exploration outside of the context of marriage resulted in stigmatization, Mabel's transgressive sexual behavior resulted in family shame.[5] In the wake of two unforeseen and devastating tragedies, Mabel ultimately took the opportunity to try to hide her shame, remaking herself as a "respectable" (i.e., "nondefective") woman. And yet just when it appeared that she may have succeeded in that reinvention, neurosyphilis—the delayed result of her previously acquired venereal disease—ended not only her second chance, but her life. Mabel's sexual transgressions intertwined with her disability, marking her as shameful in both a family and a social culture that demanded "normalcy." Having failed to redeem herself in life, she was erased in death. Mabel, her sexuality, her motherhood, and her disability vanished from both family and public memory.

Katherine Mabel Dalton

By the mid-1930s the total number of patients housed at state hospitals for the insane nationwide reached more than half a million, representing a dramatic increase from the nineteenth century.[6] For the most

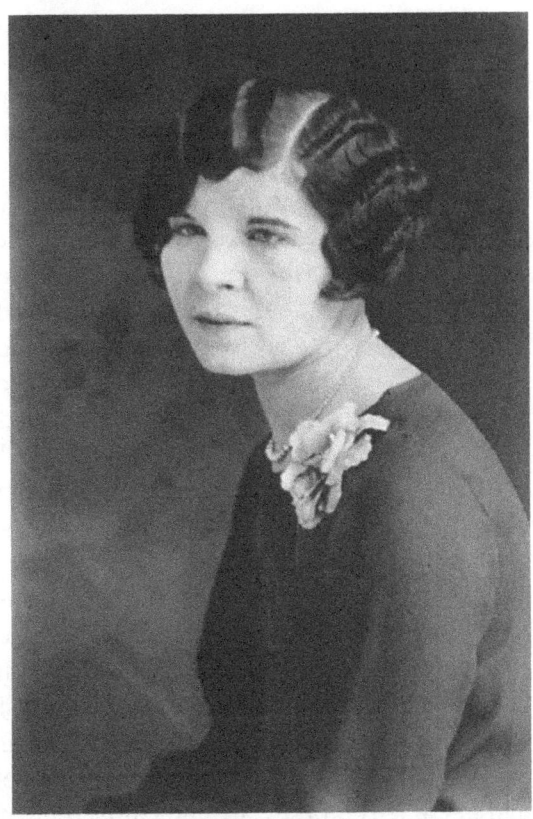

Mabel Dalton Ward Smith. Author's photo.

part, historians have had very little access to the pre-institutional life histories of these hundreds of thousands of patients, who have been lost to history because they often did not leave any recordable trace of themselves. Their erasure is a clear and direct consequence of the ways that power and inequality manifested in legal, economic, and health systems of the time.[7] In particular, housewives like Mabel rarely left tracks in the historical record, because their gendered positions as women relegated to spheres of domesticity rendered them valueless both at the time and also in the archive, leading to their erasure. As the great-niece of Mabel Smith, I have had the unique opportunity to uncover aspects of Mabel's pre-institutional life that are not always available to historians. This has meant that in addition to accessing more traditional historical sources (newspapers, census data, archival records), I have as her relative also uncovered additional tiny scraps of evidence of Mabel's early life, sometimes integrating tips and sources from genealogical research.[8] Alone, these bits of disparate information don't look like much, but stitched together they begin to flesh out a fuller picture of this particular ordinary woman, whose life ended so abruptly in disability and death. In telling her story I am recovering her voice, which was silenced first by sexual "deviance" and impairment, later by the historical processes of institutionalization and medical experimentation that labeled her disabled, and finally by the legacy of shame.[9]

Mabel Smith was born Katherine Mabel Dalton on July 3, 1902, to Michael and Katherine (Killila) Dalton of Indianapolis.[10] The first of six children, Mabel grew up in a small Irish and German Catholic community in a residential neighborhood on the southern edge of downtown. After Mabel came two more girls, Marie and Norma, followed by three boys, Raymond, Thomas, and finally Leo, born in 1920. With their daily life centered on St. John the Evangelist Catholic Church, Catholicism and Democratic Party city politics formed the neighborhood borders that shaped Mabel's and her siblings' lives. As the family grew, so did its commitment to St. John's parish, where each new baby was baptized along with the other Catholic children in the neighborhood, and Michael and Katherine also became godparents to several babies of the many relatives who lived close by. Mabel's baptism occurred on July 20, 1902, when she was still a newborn, as was the custom with Catholic infant baptism.[11] Located in the heart of downtown on West Georgia Street, St. John the Evangelist Church had become the first Catholic Church in Indianapolis in 1871, and as such, it drew in the Catholic neighbors who surrounded it, shaping their life stories across several generations.[12] As the Dalton children grew, many landmarks of their lives were carefully recorded in sacramental books at St. John's. The children can be traced from baptism to First Communion to weddings and, occasionally, to funeral services. Mabel, however, disappears from those church records much earlier than her siblings and her parents.

A son of Irish immigrants and a Democratic Party foot soldier in Indianapolis city politics, Michael Dalton won a prestigious position as city market manager in the notoriously corrupt mayor Joseph E. Bell's administration in 1914.[13] Before this elevation in city government, Michael had worked as a constable in the coroner's office while he served as Democratic Party committeeperson for the Twelfth Ward. In summer 1915 Michael was one of 128 city administrators indicted on charges of conspiracy to commit election fraud.[14] By December of that year, the charges had been dropped against Michael and 104 others due to a lack of sufficient evidence for the conspiracy charge; at the time, prosecutors noted that many of the men had indeed committed election fraud, but that they had "merely obeyed orders," and as such would not be prosecuted.[15] That said, prosecutors again filed election fraud charges against several police officers and city administrators in summer 1917. Those charges led to the convictions and resignations of six Bell supporters; despite the damning evidence presented against them, Mayor Bell responded by calling the convictions a "most regrettable affair," insisting that the convicted men "had intended to uphold the law," and suggesting that his regret lay with the judicial outcome rather than the illegal acts.[16] During the original set of indictments—the ones that included Mabel's father—Mayor Bell had arranged Michael's $5,000 bond, which he likely would not have been able to cover on his own.[17] The following year, in 1916, the Daltons left behind their rented house, having secured a new, larger house in the neighborhood, with Michael purchasing the real estate on Senate Street for $1,400.[18] Michael then equipped the new home with a telephone, at a time when only about 35 percent of American households had them.[19] The next year, in 1917, authorities charged the former controller for the Bell administration with having illicitly paid for telephone rentals for several city officers and employees in their private residences; Michael Dalton was one of those men.[20]

Despite mounting investigations into the potential criminal activity of Mayor Bell's administration, the mayor resisted any acknowledgment of wrongdoing. Instead, he repeatedly pointed to his administration's success in developing important public works projects. In addition, he claimed that religious and other community leaders regularly shared with him how pleased they were with the state of the city, which one claimed was "the cleanest that he had ever known it to be from a moral standpoint."[21] Indeed one of Bell's many accomplishments that he liked to tout was the creation of a "city vice squad" to improve the moral character of the city. This focus on "vice" and "degeneracy" as the crux of urban social problems was not unique to Indianapolis or the Bell administration. During the Progressive Era, social reformers around the nation increasingly targeted immoral and degenerate behavior as the cause of urban crime as well as social and economic ills more generally. Efforts at "cleaning up" this behavior increasingly overlapped with evolving beliefs in eugenic thinking that divided people into categories of "fit" and "unfit."[22]

As with the eugenics advocated by social reformers, the morality trumpeted by Mayor Bell and his followers resulted in sharp and exclusionary boundaries that reinforced existing power inequalities. In the political context, it appears that Mayor Bell and his administration enriched themselves as they supposedly spruced up the morality of the city. From the posting of bond to the purchase of real estate and the funding of a telephone, Michael Dalton and his family seem to have financially benefited from their association with the Bell administration. But in the wake of that association, they saw their relative good fortune decline. Catapulted into the middle class during Bell's time in office, the Dalton family had by 1920 returned to the laboring class, with Michael resuming wage work, becoming first a machine operator, then a clerk for the automobile industry, and finally a carpenter.[23] Nonetheless, the Daltons' brief flirtation with political power was enough to secure their future. Even though he lost political and economic standing in the aftermath of the Bell administration, Michael's temporary foray into city government and politics still resulted in the purchase of a home, which ultimately elevated the Daltons into a previously unattainable position of financial security, one that allowed them to enjoy the comforts of a newly middle-classed America, at least temporarily.

During those high-flying years, as Mabel grew into a teenager, she chafed against the restrictions of her small world, the expectations of her parents' Catholicism, and perhaps, too, her father's increasingly public profile in a city administration dedicated to rooting out vice. In 1922, just after she turned twenty, Mabel found herself pregnant and unmarried.[24] Her boyfriend, Charles Irvin Ward (called Jack Poole by his friends), lived near Mabel's family home.[25] It seems likely that the two met in the neighborhood when they were quite young and both families lived briefly on Chadwick Street.[26] Although the Dalton family's purchase of the home on Senate Street meant that Mabel moved two miles away from Irvin, the new distance likely posed little challenge, both because of the popular and widely used electric streetcar, and because working-class youth increasingly socialized outside of the neighborhood at dance halls, nickelodeons, and other commercialized spaces.[27] As scholars have previously noted, these new nighttime commercial amusements created a "heterosocial environment" that "encouraged a new sexual ethic among working-class youth."[28] It seems quite likely that Mabel and Irvin took advantage of this emerging social scene, experimenting with both public leisure and sexual exploration.

Mabel's unwed pregnancy made public her private sexual transgressions, and the resulting shame demanded a resolution. As with city politicians concerned about vice, Catholic leaders and local Catholic parishioners supported a heterosexual nuclear family, worrying that immorality and transgressive sexual behavior threatened that structure.[29] Irvin Ward was likely not Catholic, and he was almost certainly not part of the Daltons' plan for their firstborn daughter. In February 1923, twenty-year-old Mabel and twenty-two-year-old Irvin married in a civil ceremony. They moved into a residence in the neighborhood at 827 South West Street, and Irvin worked as a "pool room keeper," while Mabel stopped working for wages outside the home. A mere week after their wedding, on February 27, Mabel Ward gave birth to a baby boy at their home.[30] Although it is difficult to know how Mabel's parents felt about her unwed pregnancy and the rushed civil ceremony, it seems highly likely that the situation created conflict between Mabel and her parents. In the early decades of the twentieth century, working-class parents in particular feared the close association of nighttime socializing, premarital sex, and prostitution.[31] Shame and censure (or fear of these) likely shaped Mabel's parents' response to her unwed pregnancy. Shame—and the threat of being shamed—has historically functioned as a social mechanism for establishing and enforcing the norms and behaviors deemed acceptable by a community.[32] Perhaps Michael and Katherine stopped talking to their daughter, cutting her off from their Catholic sphere; or perhaps they were the ones who insisted on the wedding, in the hopes of keeping their daughter somewhat connected to that Catholic sphere. At the time, Katherine still had five children under the age of eighteen, with the three youngest all under the age of twelve, so perhaps her time and attention were taken up with the demands of child-rearing and other domestic duties. Whatever Mabel's parents' exact feelings may have been, shame likely affected their interactions with their oldest daughter. Unlike the future weddings of her siblings, Mabel's wedding was not recorded at St. John the Evangelist Church. It seems especially likely that for a Catholic family enmeshed in this Catholic neighborhood and culture, an unwed pregnancy and rushed civil marriage would have prompted scorn, shame, or silence. Or perhaps all three. What is abundantly clear is that nobody in the family ever talked about Mabel's pregnancy or her son.

Two tragedies occurred during Mabel's young married life that provide health history clues suggesting the origins of Mabel's syphilis infection, even as they also prompted the unintended backdrop against which Mabel sought to remake herself into a respectable woman. The first tragedy occurred on the same late February day that Mabel birthed her baby boy. Nearly immediately after his birth, Mabel lost her child. Born alive at their home at 11:10 a.m., Mabel and Irvin's baby boy died five minutes later.[33] Although the cause of death was not recorded, hindsight and all available evidence point compellingly toward congenital syphilis, a common outcome for babies of syphilis-infected mothers. Although it is very possible that neither Mabel nor Irvin knew about their syphilis infections at this point, the following year another tragedy occurred, contributing even more evidence suggestive of syphilis. Less than a year after their infant boy died in their home, Irvin died in the very same house of a cerebral hemorrhage. Surviving records do not mention neurosyphilis, but cerebral hemorrhage—especially in an otherwise healthy young man—is highly suggestive of the diagnosis, just as the infant's early death similarly hints at congenital syphilis infection.[34] Within a year's time, twenty-two-year-old Mabel had lost everything, and yet the worst was yet to come. She had no idea that she, too, had been infected with syphilis; six years later, shortly after she married her second husband, Arthur Smith, that silent syphilis infection roared to life.

During the six years between Irvin's death and Mabel's admission to CSH, the details of Mabel's life come in and out of focus. We know that at some point in the aftermath of Irvin's death Mabel moved back to the Dalton family home on Senate Street. From 1926 to 1928 she worked as a stenographer.[35] Perhaps she helped bring her sister Norma into the same line of work, because in the 1930 census Norma (still living on Senate Street at the time) was similarly employed as a stenographer.[36] On February 6, 1929, Mabel's sister Marie, who was closest to her in age, married James Cormack at St. John's. The groomsman was a man named Arthur Smith.[37] Was this how Mabel came to be introduced to her second husband? Did she meet Arthur through her sister Marie? It seems likely, and yet, perhaps somewhat mysteriously, Mabel did not serve as Marie's bridesmaid; instead, their younger sister, Norma, filled this role. Perhaps the shame of Mabel's past sexual transgression kept her from serving in this more public and celebratory role.[38] Mabel is not mentioned in any of the wedding records, and yet, despite her apparent absence from her sister's church wedding, Mabel Dalton Ward married Arthur Smith just eight months later, presumably in another civil ceremony. Arthur, who was three years older than Mabel, was a fellow St. John's parishioner who held a steady job as a plumber's helper.[39]

In October 1929, then, Mabel attempted married life anew with Arthur. She was older and had suffered significant loss. But now (at least perhaps from her parents' view) she was back on track toward becoming a respectable woman. To this end, either Mabel or Arthur (or perhaps both) lied to census workers, reporting that Mabel's marriage to Arthur was her first, and that her age at first marriage was twenty-seven.[40] Mabel's past life—her unwed pregnancy at the age of twenty, her experience of childbirth, the sudden death of her baby, the loss of her young husband—all of it, was erased. Mabel and Arthur's marriage in 1929 began the process of rewriting a life, constructing a narrative that better conformed to the expectations for young, able-bodied white women in the 1920s. Maybe they felt hopeful. Maybe Mabel had collaborated in the rewriting of her story. Maybe she hoped to put her past behind her. Maybe the experience of having been shamed motivated her own intentional forgetting of the pain. Or perhaps Mabel continued to feel deep grief and loss in the wake of the deaths she had experienced. Whatever her thoughts and feelings upon her second marriage, Mabel was almost certainly not aware of the syphilis infection that had taken hold within her. Nor could she have anticipated the painful ways that that syphilis infection would refuse to let her move on.

Syphilis in Indianapolis: Shifting Cultural Norms and Venereal Disease

In the post–World War I period of the 1920s, Indianapolis, like many northern cities in the nation, was shaped by extreme nativism and racism coupled with a swift backlash against "modern" notions of gender. Xenophobic fears about the world led to isolationist sentiment and a renewed effort at maintaining restrictive gender and race norms, despite, or perhaps because of, the changing demographics of urban spaces. If the prewar period saw the ascendance of white European immigrant communities in the Midwest, the postwar period witnessed a quickening of the assimilation of those communities into something more akin to white American.[41] Those European immigrant communities had been instrumental in supporting an idealized sense of morality shaped by Christian religious beliefs. Thus, even as European immigrant communities were encouraged to assimilate, their highly gendered expectations for and about women, men, and sex dominated the cultural sphere in the 1920s.[42] Indeed, the postwar cultural backlash that gave rise to the growing nativism and racism also prompted a moral panic regarding the behavior and purity of young "liberated" women.[43] Thus, even as "shame culture" had somewhat dissipated by the mid-nineteenth century, the reliance on shame to enforce certain expectations about sexual propriety and morality persisted deep into the 1920s in several regions within the United States, including Indiana.[44] Social anxieties about shifting gender boundaries and sexual behaviors, coupled with the persistence of shame and shaming, mapped onto cultural concerns about the materialism wrought by the burgeoning consumer culture and the vice it spawned to induce a new moral panic that was particularly evident in Indiana.

One important example of the shame-fueled moral panic of the 1920s can be found in the work of the husband-and-wife sociologist team Robert and Helen Lynd, who arrived in the heartland from the East Coast during the 1920s to study Muncie, Indiana, in their quest to understand and interpret cultural change. The culmination of their research, the 1929 volume *Middletown*, highlighted the social stigma attached to women who transgressed sexual boundaries in the 1920s. "A heavy taboo," wrote the Lynds, "supported by law and by both religious and popular sanctions, rests upon sexual relationships between persons who are not married." The stigma resulted in more consequences for women than for men, as evidenced by the language used to describe both. Noting a slight shift in men's perspectives, one interviewee, described by the Lynds as a "young buck about town in the eighties," stated that "the fellows nowadays don't seem to mind being seen on the street with a fast woman."[45] The Lynds also noted that although "houses of prostitution" appeared to be fewer in the 1920s than in the 1890s, "a comparison ... on this point is fruitless, because as the judge of the juvenile court points out, 'the automobile has become a house of prostitution on wheels.'"[46] Cars provided newfound privacy for the flourishing of illicit sexual encounters, prompting significant social anxiety. Consumer cultural shifts, which encompassed this widespread availability of the automobile, had reduced every woman with access to a car either to a potential sexual threat or to a potential victim of sexual aggression.[47] *Middletown* revealed a larger cultural fear that saw sex, consumer culture, and vice as integrally connected.[48]

Meanwhile, in Indianapolis—just over sixty miles southwest of Muncie, but with ten times its 1920 population—public leaders similarly found themselves concerned about the confluence of the shifting consumer culture, women, and sex.[49] A 1929 survey financed by the Indianapolis Foundation (the major philanthropic community association in the city) and conducted by the Council of Social Agencies reported on the leisure activities of the people of Indianapolis, noting that "through the ages the people have striven for time which they could call their own, time in which they could invite their souls and indulge themselves in the things they yearned to do.... But up to comparatively recent times only a few achieved leisure while the masses continued to struggle for it. Now, however, it can be asserted that not only a few but the many have it and they have it in abundance."[50] Concern over the potential "misuse" of this newfound abundant leisure time, which characterized many of the report's findings, suggests a pervasive anxiety about cultural change in the 1920s. In his disability history of institutionalized women, Michael Rembis notes that "defectiveness" was constructed to include women who "misused" their leisure. Indeed, "sexually delinquent" women were broadly associated with mental "defectiveness" and "feeblemindedness" and, as a result, institutionally segregated from the larger society.[51] Mistrust of working women's ability to "properly" manage their leisure time shaped the very meanings of mental disability in the 1920s.

Social concerns about the proper usage of leisure time reflected a broader worry about the potential impact of transgressive behavior on "healthy" minds and conceptions of "normalcy." Survey author Eugene T. Lies listed several "types of misuse," which included "idling, meandering, gambling, trash-reading, razzy-jazzy joy-riding, illicit sex-practices, marauding, bad gang activities, over-indulgence in mere amusements," and "recreation of the wrong kind, in the wrong places and at wrong times."[52] Ultimately Lies and the survey committee worried not only about individual deviance, but also about the consequences of this perceived "defectiveness" on the larger community and its ability to provide essential services. This line of thinking echoed that of the increasingly pervasive eugenic ideology that shaped reform movements and medicine in the interwar era.[53] As Lies noted, the potential consequences of individual immorality included the "breakdown of ambition, of health, of efficiency, and therefore of earning power, degrading of tastes and moral stamina, delinquency and crime," all of which ultimately required intervention by the "doctor, nurse, hospital, social hygienist, psychiatrist," and so forth.[54] Directly linking degeneracy to health-care resources and costs, Lies urged early social intervention.[55] This stance was not entirely unlike that of the previous decade's mayoral administration, with its fixation on vice and morality, though Lies and the committee relied on social scientific methods rather than political graft. But ultimately the social scientists, too, drew connections between proper behavior, morality, and "good" health.

Lies and the survey committee recommended frequent physical activity in nature to make good use of leisure time and thwart any temptations toward "misuse." As examples of healthier leisure choices from earlier decades, the report included some respondents' recollections of their childhood, a time that would have spanned 1890–1910. One survey respondent, a young woman, recalled co-ed bicycling parties in which "boys and girls would bike all day up to Broad Ripple and then have breakfast." She continued, "We came back from such trips tired, dirty, happy. Did the neighbors talk? I should say they did . . . they could see the young people going to ruination, but mothers were wise then, as they are today."[56] The survey authors seemed to imply that although an earlier generation of adults may have similarly fretted about cultural change, at least the young people "going to ruination" at that time were headed there on bicycles. Social reformers of the 1920s worried by contrast that automobiles, which removed young people from nature and, more importantly, provided them with unprecedented privacy for sexual experimentation, had become the modern physical site for "misuse" of leisure. Indeed, the report noted a 184 percent increase in passenger cars in Indianapolis over the course of the decade. As Lies wrote, "We learned that there is one passenger car for every four persons in Marion County."[57] And just as the Lynds' respondents in *Middletown* lamented, the automobile promoted all sorts of vice. From the automobile to illicit sex, straight to the insane asylum, the new leisure opportunities of the 1920s seemed to change—and threaten—everything.[58]

Social anxieties about deviant sexual behavior typically targeted young women as the source of the troublesome immorality. An *Indianapolis News* article reported that one of the most "exclusive streets in the city" (North Meridian) had been "invaded" by "bobbed-haired, bare-headed . . . women soliciting nefariously."[59] This focus on women's behavior as the root cause of immorality was of course nothing new. As several historians have noted, most of the federally supported anti-syphilis efforts during World War I similarly targeted women (both prostitutes and women viewed as promiscuous) as agents of venereal disease, with male soldiers their unwitting victims.[60] The venereal disease policy of the wartime Commission on Training Camp Activities (CTCA), which ultimately sought to protect *soldiers* from *girls*, who were increasingly viewed as the source of the syphilis threat, resulted in the incarceration of tens of thousands of young women in federally financed detention centers. Without trials or due process, isolating and imprisoning women accused of sex offenses became the major policy response to the public health threat of syphilis.[61] Within this larger context it is perhaps not surprising that in the wake of the Great War, women continued to be singled out for scorn. Shame and embarrassment associated with a syphilis diagnosis permeated this postwar period, and women were particularly vulnerable to accusations of immorality.[62] Although they made up a minority of the paretic patients at CSH, women with neurosyphilis—both white and Black—experienced intertwining forms of social stigma that labeled them disabled as well as gender defective.

These deeply rooted community concerns regarding immoral sexual behavior overlapped with the transitions taking place in syphilis prevention efforts as well as shifts in psychiatry more broadly. Although psychiatrists and state mental institutions increasingly looked to laboratory science in determining causes of insanity in the early twentieth century, community leaders, reformers, and other public advocates often continued to emphasize immorality as a primary cause.[63] Determining the causes of mental troubles was contested terrain. Even as psychiatry staked a claim in medical science, eugenic ideology animating that science created a through line from the earlier beliefs about immorality to the more modern science-based explanations that used heredity to establish "normality" and "abnormality."[64] Increasingly embracing these eugenic explanations of illness, reformers and psychiatrists alike worried publicly that mental and physical impairments that required serious medical and psychiatric intervention not only threatened the individual, but dangerously overtaxed the community's precious resources.

In their efforts at containing this perceived threat of "degeneracy," asylum leaders and reformers hoped the economic cost-saving argument might motivate action and support on the part of state governments, and nowhere was this more apparent than in Indiana.[65] In a 1917 speech at a statewide health conference, Dr. Max Bahr noted that the care and treatment of the insane cost the state of Indiana $10 million per year and that the successful prevention of syphilis would reduce this yearly cost by $2 million.[66] The Indiana Committee on Mental Defectives championed a version of this economic argument five years later, in a report to the governor: "It is a conservative estimate that today the care in state institutions of those directly wrecked by syphilis costs Indiana over one-third of one million dollars a year; while those in these institutions suffering indirectly from this disease cost the state a much larger amount."[67] A commitment to eugenics and the desire to limit the community impact of those deemed "unfit" shaped both the creation of this Indiana committee and its conclusions, which it disseminated in reports issued in 1916, 1918, and 1922. Indeed, the committee worked directly with the Eugenics Record Office (ERO), with proponents of eugenics exhibiting a strong influence on its work.[68] Through its reform recommendations, the committee's 1922 report revealed prejudicial stereotypes about crime, vice, and madness. The authors worried extensively about "the influx of undesirable citizens," whom they referred to as "shiftless, 'do-less,' 'no-account' people," and recommended, among other things, that the state should "assist in every way in the operation of the Federal anti-vice law now in force."[69] Ultimately, the committee members, who advocated for the reasonably humane treatment of the mad (they "condemned" the common practice of holding people experiencing mental troubles in jails), nonetheless blamed them for their impairments. Acknowledging that a "large proportion of cases of mental defect of all varieties is due directly to syphilis, alcohol, and habit-forming drugs," the committee hoped to engage the state in a more forceful and aggressive crackdown on the behaviors that led to these vices.[70] Although these advocates hoped to end paretic insanity, their approach to prevention, which relied on eugenic ideology, reinforced the very stereotypes that stigmatized and shamed those suffering from the disease.

The ongoing tension between public health advocates' desire to stem the spread of syphilis through community education and the deeply entrenched social taboo associated with venereal disease played itself out in local community leaders' thwarted attempts to build a relationship with national activists. As early as 1927, the Indianapolis Foundation committed to funding a city survey to be conducted by the American Social Hygiene Association (ASHA), a national organization with significant venereal disease campaign experience and personnel to conduct urban surveys in the fight against syphilis. Despite the promise of funding in 1927 and again every year for the next five years, political opposition on the part of the president of the Indianapolis Board of Health prevented the study from taking place.[71] In a 1932 letter from Bascom Johnson of ASHA to Eugene Foster, director of the Indianapolis Foundation, Johnson encouraged Foster to maintain his commitment to supporting citywide anti-syphilis efforts, despite the political challenges. With considerable experience in ASHA's long-standing efforts to fight syphilis, Johnson had spent the World War I years leading the CTCA's campaign, which targeted prostitution and alcohol as culprits.[72] Thus it is perhaps not surprising that fourteen years later in his communications with Indianapolis civic leaders Johnson continued to focus his efforts on the threats to Indianapolis residents posed by commercialized prostitution, writing, "May we suggest that it is important for you and the other socially minded citizens of your city to know whether your growing boys and girls are being subjected to the influences described above."[73] But despite Johnson's support, Foster's hands were tied. "It seems a pity," wrote Dr. Walter Clarke, also of ASHA, "that with the fund available and the local leaders . . . and others interested in the project that it should be held up on account of the opposition of the President of the Board of Health."[74] But that is exactly what occurred.

In part the problem lay with the structure of the Indianapolis Board of Health, membership of which changed with each incoming mayoral administration. This led to inconsistent and ever-changing health policy, which posed even more challenges for the city's anti-syphilis efforts. Indeed, during the late 1920s and early 1930s under the leadership of Dr. Frederick Jackson, who seemed disinterested in anti-syphilis efforts, the Indianapolis Board of Health opposed the Indianapolis Foundation's financial offer to fund the venereal disease survey. Meanwhile, the Indianapolis Board of Health oversaw operations and policies at City Hospital, the hospital that was often the first line of defense in triaging and treating late-stage syphilis, and the hospital to which Mabel Smith, like so many others, was first taken when she began showing signs of madness.[75]

Despite the Indianapolis Board of Health's opposition to the citywide venereal disease survey, the Indianapolis Foundation nonetheless found ways to fund anti-syphilis and mental treatment efforts. Perhaps most importantly, under Foster's leadership, the Indianapolis Foundation provided financial support to City Hospital. First, the foundation paid to help establish a psychiatric ward at the hospital. In 1925 Foster hired and paid (through the foundation) Mrs. May D. Ballou as a psychiatric social worker at City Hospital. A professional social worker with extensive experience treating madness, Mrs. Ballou had formerly been a social worker with Hull-House in Chicago. The recruitment and retention of Mrs. Ballou demonstrated the Indianapolis Foundation's commitment to professionalization of City Hospital's chaotic attempts at dealing with insanity. In addition, in 1929 the foundation conducted a study that uncovered several problems, particularly in the admitting department, that led to inefficiency and chaos at the hospital; responding to these problems, the foundation hired two professional women, Miss Catherine Sadlier and Miss Lucy Clare Finley, to restructure and run the admissions department, even paying their salaries for the year 1930 until they could be covered by City Hospital's internal budget. The Indianapolis Foundation also regularly provided grants to City Hospital's venereal disease clinic to "pay for car fare and other incidentals that might prevent clients from coming in."[76] Thus, city politics notwithstanding, the foundation's leaders, clearly concerned about the public

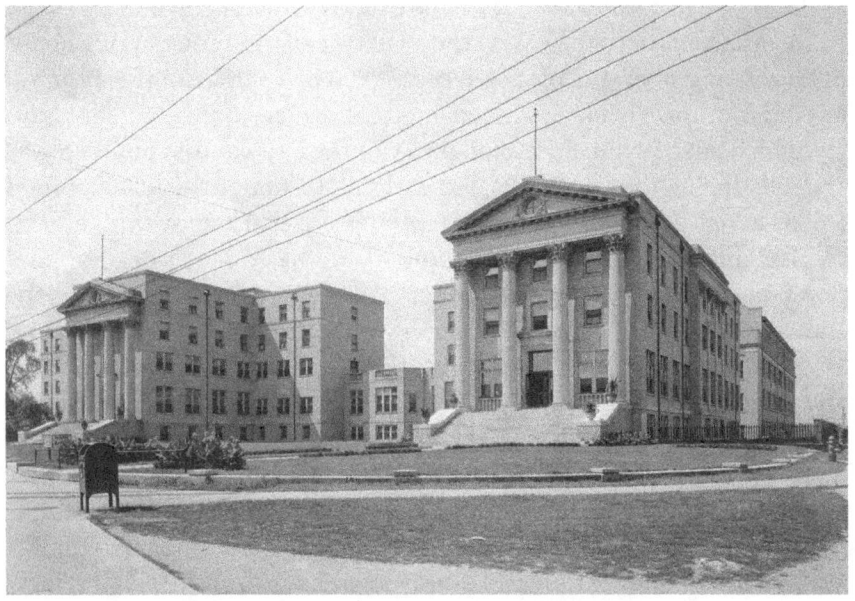

Indianapolis City Hospital, August 1927. Bass Photo Company Collection. Courtesy of the Indiana Historical Society.

health threat posed by syphilis, found ways to fund constructive efforts at prevention and treatment for some of the city's most vulnerable.

Before 1925, Indiana residents who sought medical care for early-stage syphilis could be treated with Salvarsan (an organic arsenic compound that was distributed as a yellow powder that had to be mixed with liquid prior to injection) or Neosalvarsan (an updated version of the compound that was supposedly easier to apply).[77] Unfortunately, neither treatment proved effective for those suffering from neurosyphilis. Once insanity began to show itself, family members often sought care at City Hospital. Such was the case for Mabel; her husband, Arthur, checked her into City Hospital when she became inexplicably "maniacal." Despite its foundation-supported psychopathic ward, City Hospital nonetheless lacked the funding, expertise, and resources for the long-term care and treatment of paresis in neurosyphilis patients. And yet overcrowding and underfunding at CSH meant that very often paretic patients waited for weeks or even months in local hospitals or county jails for space to become available for their transfer. Mabel stayed at City Hospital relatively briefly, arriving in September 1930 and transferring to CSH the next month. As Dr. Tidwell noted in her CSH patient file, Mabel had become "suddenly" incoherent and confused.[78] Many paretic patients experienced this sudden onset of insanity and paralysis, although others experienced a gradual onset of symptoms, until the point at which the insanity overtook their daily lives and family members had no choice but to send them away. Regardless of the duration or onset history of symptoms, patient files are replete with lengthy descriptions of the painful and humiliating manner in which insanity overtook ill patients.

Women, Gender, and Madness at CSH: The Interwar Period

When Mabel arrived at CSH, she was just one in a long line of women who had been or were later to be institutionalized. First conceived of by an 1844 act of the Indiana General Assembly, which determined to build a "state lunatic asylum," the Indianapolis Hospital for the Insane—as it was initially named—took several years to be constructed and become ready for operation. The national reformer Dorothea Dix traveled to Indiana in order to lobby for the funding of the institution, and in summer 1845 the state purchased farmland about four miles south of downtown to become the site of the asylum. After a series of legislative funding delays and construction challenges, the Indianapolis Hospital for the Insane opened its doors in November 1848.[79] One of the first among a wave of openings of state asylums across the country, the Indianapolis Hospital for the Insane embarked on its own long and controversial history of care and treatment of patients deemed "insane" in the state of Indiana. From 1870 to 1936 the total number of patients hospitalized in insane asylums across the nation increased exponentially, from 45,000 to 566,000, with CSH experiencing similar expansive growth.[80]

Perhaps the most famous woman patient at CSH, Anna Agnew, predated Mabel's incarceration by about forty years. A married mother of four who spent seven years institutionalized for insanity, from 1878 to 1885, Mrs. Agnew (as she was called and also referred to herself) wrote a memoir of her experience that was published in 1886.[81] Agnew recorded her attempted suicides, her recurring thoughts of suicide, the many abuses she suffered at CSH, her deteriorating relationship with her husband (who accused her of having intentionally hidden her insanity from him upon their marriage), and her positive relationship with a woman physician at CSH, Dr. Sarah Stockton.[82] Unlike Agnew, with her late nineteenth-century medical incarceration, Mabel Smith experienced CSH during a decidedly different historical moment, one in which eugenic thinking influenced modern medical explanations for insanity, even as a desire to solve the problems posed by this insanity prompted experimentation with increasingly more radical therapies.

Historians of women's institutionalization have documented the ways that labeling women "insane" and "mentally defective" has at least in part resulted from historically and socially constructed gendered expectations about women's proper behavior. The naming of women as "deviant" has itself been a process of historical construction shaped by the changing rhetoric embedded in medicine and psychiatry as well as the many cultural shifts that occurred during the interwar era.[83] The shame and shaming that accompanied such labels were ultimately meant to induce conformity, leaving women isolated and alone.[84] From the mid-nineteenth century up through the middle of the twentieth century, women's institutionalization often reflected the power and inequality inherent in the gendered expectations of both womanhood and good mental health; in other words, many institutionalized women were labeled as "mad," "defective," or "deviant" for failing to live up to these gendered expectations. Social and asylum labeling functioned to exert power and control over women.[85] Thus, historically, women who have broken gender norms have been at particular risk of being labeled "mad."

Somewhat in contrast, Mabel's story engages an experience of acquired mental and physical impairment and death caused by a biologically documented disease. Although Mabel, too, transgressed gender norms by engaging in a premarital sexual relationship, her "madness" and her medical incarceration resulted directly from a somatic illness. In some ways, then, the larger body of literature on the gendered dimension of insanity and institutionalization fails to account for Mabel's embodied experience of madness. This is where feminist disability history becomes particularly helpful in illuminating the lived experience of Mabel and women like her.[86] Examining the historical context of women's experience and treatment of neurosyphilis allows for wrestling with the lived experience of physical and mental impairment. Although at the time researchers and physicians believed that neurosyphilis afflicted men far more commonly than women, prompting them to generally discuss the illness in gendered terms as a man's disease, in reality Mabel and many other women like her suffered and died from neurosyphilis.[87] Women's erasure from that story both in the moment and in historical reflection has led to a lack of critical inquiry regarding their lived disabilities and the gendered constructions of their experiences. It has also hidden their individual experiences of shame and shaming for their embodied experiences of sexuality, reproduction, and disability.[88]

As institutionalizations increased during the interwar era (with syphilis accounting for at least 20 percent of new admissions and schizophrenia prompting an additional 22 percent), the field of psychiatry continued to grow, defining itself at least in part on the biological basis of madness.[89] At CSH, Mabel likely found herself in the company of many other patients who also suffered from neurosyphilis, acquiring both mental and physical impairments that had wordlessly moved them from the category of fit to "unfit." Hoping to cure women and men of these illnesses while simultaneously saving the community from the economic impact of their disabilities, doctors at state asylums began experimenting with insulin shock treatment, electroconvulsive treatment, and, of course, malaria therapy.[90] Mabel's stay at CSH coincided with this period of experimentation and radical therapeutic intervention. Her experience of malaria therapy treatment, which failed to offer her its promised cure, entirely shaped her experience of institutionalization, especially in the last few weeks of her life. Unlike Anna Agnew, who was eventually discharged, Mabel Smith experienced no improvement at CSH. Rather, Mabel died at the institution six weeks after being inoculated with malaria. As such, Mabel Smith's treatment and death at CSH were inextricably connected to the work of its lead pathologist and director of research, Dr. Walter L. Bruetsch.

CHAPTER 2

Dr. Walter L. Bruetsch

In fall 1930 Dr. Walter L. Bruetsch, the lead pathologist of the Central State Hospital (CSH) in Indianapolis, Indiana, and a newly minted American citizen, was preparing for a six-month leave from CSH and the United States. With five years of the malaria therapy experiment under his belt in Indianapolis, he and Dr. Max Bahr, superintendent of the state facility, had already published and presented their initial findings throughout the country. Now, Bruetsch was ready to take his work international, back home to Germany. And so, for the first time since his arrival in the States, Bruetsch prepared for an extended stay in Europe, where he intended to continue presenting and discussing his research work.[1] Preoccupied with trip planning as he surely was, Bruetsch may very well have paid little attention to Mabel Smith, the young paretic patient with the crossed eyes who was transferred over from City Hospital in October of that year. While Bruetsch, who was a mere six years older than Mabel, prepared for his worldly travels, Mabel began the very small and confined last chapter of her short life. When Mabel died in February 1931, just a few weeks after her injection with malaria, it was not Bruetsch who certified her death, but rather Dr. Francis Prenatti, another CSH physician; by the time Mabel drew her last breath, Bruetsch had already set out for Germany to promote his malaria therapy research.

Dr. Bruetsch's experimental work remade CSH into a major center for biomedical research, and the malaria therapy treatment of neurosyphilis both laid the foundation for this shift and became the crown jewel of the program. The disabled minds and bodies of women and men incarcerated at CSH made this research and its resulting professional prestige possible, though this fact was unacknowledged by either Dr. Bruetsch or Superintendent Bahr. In their overarching desire to "cure" insanity, Bruetsch and Bahr injected malaria into hundreds of women and men suffering from severe mental and physical impairment.[2] As with other mentally disabled women and men at CSH, Mabel's insanity, treatment, and death were ultimately overseen by Bruetsch. And although Mabel Smith and Walter Bruetsch most likely did not know each other—Bruetsch himself did not sign any of Mabel's patient records—they were nevertheless linked by their positions as patient and doctor within an institutional context of research and treatment that prioritized "cure" over all else.[3] During her stay at CSH, Mabel's already diminished mental and physical health declined so rapidly that even if she had met Bruetsch, she likely would not have remembered such an encounter, and likewise, by the time that Mabel was injected with malaria in January 1931, Bruetsch had seen hundreds of patients before her and quite like her. Most certainly preoccupied with his upcoming six-month journey to Germany, Bruetsch would scarcely have noticed or remembered any potential encounters with Mabel. And yet, they played critical, if unequal, roles in each other's lives, one providing the experimental treatment, the other becoming the scientific data.

Drs. Max Bahr and Walter L. Bruetsch

Superintendent Max Bahr recruited Dr. Walter L. Bruetsch from Germany to CSH in a concerted effort to prioritize research and medical progress based on scientific experimentation. Together, Superintendent Bahr and Dr. Bruetsch began the malaria therapy project at CSH in 1925 and kept it running for more than two decades. And together, Superintendent Bahr and Dr. Bruetsch collected and treated over a thousand neurosyphilis patients with malaria, even as they built an enormous research database, in the process positioning CSH and its growing pathology department as a prominent national site for biomedical research. Bahr pinned his hopes for a cure to the neurosyphilis crisis and for a modernized and globally renowned research center at CSH on the young German researcher. Over the course of several decades, the pair worked to make both dreams happen; a steady supply of patients marginalized by disability and shame made it possible.

The two doctors' life stories intersected at the crossroads of psychiatry, medical experimentation, and the increasing American interest in laboratory research in the aftermath of the Great War.[4] Max Bahr had first arrived at CSH in 1898, by way of Washington, DC, where he had served as chief resident physician of the Government Emergency Hospital. While in DC, he had several times visited Saint Elizabeths Hospital, the federal insane asylum. These visits had endeared him to the idea of working in psychiatry. During his time at CSH, Dr. Bahr discovered that German psychiatry seemed far more advanced than the US medical specialty, and he hoped to help modernize psychiatric practices at CSH. With his curiosity and interest growing, Bahr was granted a leave of absence to work and learn at the Charité Hospital in Berlin under "the tutelage of one of the foremost psychiatrists in Europe," as Bahr later remembered it.[5] At the time, German medical researchers stood at the forefront of connecting insanity to physical illness. Indeed, from 1870 to 1914, Germany was the destination for physicians around the globe who hoped to take on advanced training in a variety of clinical medical specialties, including psychiatry. As many as fifteen thousand American-born physicians embarked on postgraduate study and training

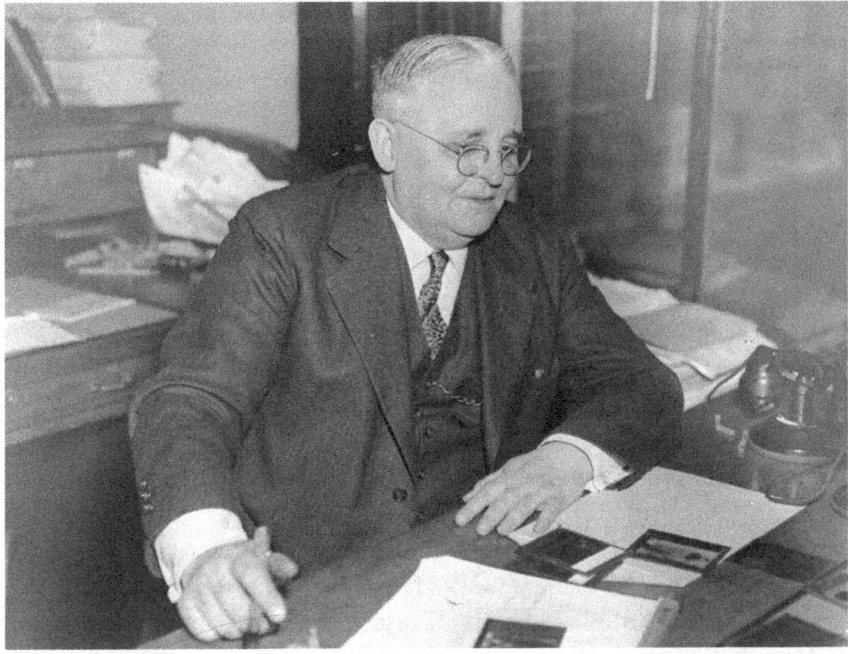

Superintendent Max Bahr, MD. Central State Hospital Collection, 2006071, neg. 044.tif. Courtesy of the Indiana State Archives.

in Germany prior to the Great War.[6] In making the trek to Germany, Bahr became just one of the many motivated physicians who made their way to German universities in order to study the brain.[7]

Back at CSH in his role as a physician, Dr. Bahr noted that nearly 20 percent of patients confined to the Indianapolis hospital between 1908 and 1916 suffered from syphilis.[8] Overwhelmed by the extent of this biological cause of insanity, Bahr felt an urgent need to respond to this public health crisis.[9] In spring 1923 the board of trustees appointed Dr. Bahr acting superintendent of CSH, and the following year in the wake of the death of his predecessor, Dr. George F. Edenharter, who had served in the position for thirty years, Bahr assumed the role of superintendent. In this new leadership position, Superintendent Bahr focused on expanding research and teaching as a centerpiece of the work of CSH.[10] Noting that his predecessor's construction of one of the first "pathological laboratories" devoted to scientific research in psychiatry had created the conditions for CSH to house hundreds of "interesting and instructive gross neurological specimens," Dr. Bahr used his first annual report as superintendent to recommit the hospital to becoming a first-class site for research, investigation, and teaching in the "Science of Mental and Nervous Diseases."[11] Like many psychiatrists at the time, Bahr hoped to elevate psychiatry to the realm of medical science through cutting-edge research and treatments that promised to cure insanity.

Drawing on his extensive knowledge and experience of modern German psychiatric research, Superintendent Bahr immediately sought out Dr. Bruetsch to join him in this endeavor as CSH's lead pathologist. Dr. Walter L. Bruetsch was born in Germany on November 25, 1896. As a teenager he attended gymnasium in Heidelberg, excelling in Latin before serving in the First World War. A lieutenant in the German infantry, Bruetsch suffered a spinal cord injury at the Battle of the Somme, leaving him temporarily paralyzed from the waist down. Treated by a French neurosurgeon, Bruetsch regained the use of his legs. He channeled his own experience of traumatic injury into a career in medicine, earning his medical degree in 1922.[12] Bruetsch then trained with the famed Julius Wagner-Jauregg, who had popularized malaria fever therapy. On February 13, 1924, twenty-seven-year-old Bruetsch arrived in Philadelphia from Hamburg.[13] From there he made his way to Marion County, Indiana, where he spent much of his life and career as lead pathologist and medical researcher.[14]

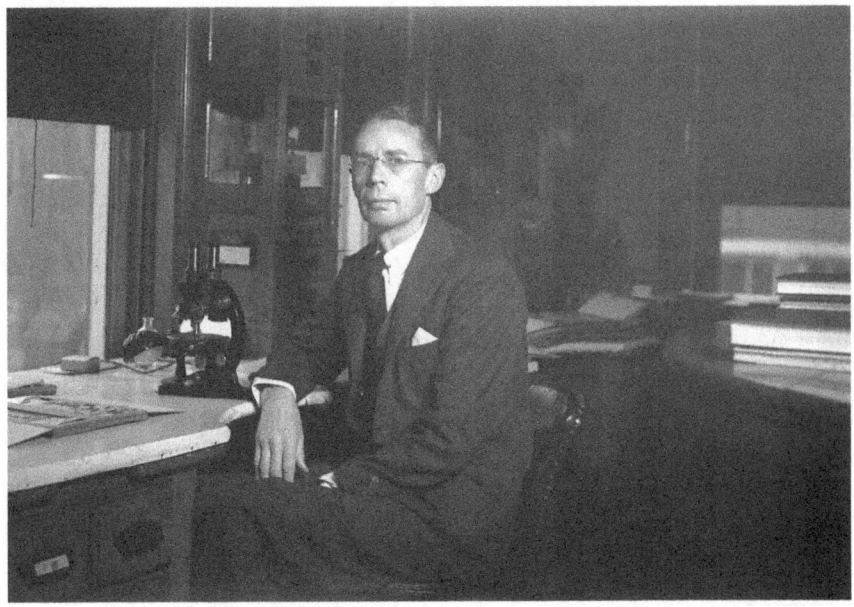

Walter L. Bruetsch, MD. Central State Hospital Collection, 2006071, neg. 001.tif. Courtesy of the Indiana State Archives.

Walter Bruetsch, like other German medical doctors and researchers of the 1920s, was fully committed to laboratory experimentation in the service of medical progress. Bahr identified Bruetsch, with his knowledge, experience, and willingness to experiment, as the most important piece of the curative puzzle for the problem of neurosyphilis that plagued CSH.[15] The many American physician-students who had traveled to Germany for advanced study and research returned home committed to scientific experimentation.[16] For psychiatrists, this increasingly meant experimenting with radical therapies that relied on the assumption that physical illness caused mental troubles.[17] Operating as they were within the wider context of a growing medical and public health embrace of eugenic thinking, leaders like Bahr hoped that medical research and experimentation might proffer a solution to the financial strain that state mental institutions placed on local communities and states.[18] Responding both to the pressures of this local context and to the more global cultural desire to keep up with German progress, Bahr and Bruetsch became key figures in this process at CSH. Perhaps one of the most important selling points about Dr. Bruetsch was his experience working with the founder of malaria therapy, the famed Julius Wagner-Jauregg.

Neurosyphilis and Malaria Therapy

Early twentieth-century medical advances importantly established a biological cause for syphilis-induced insanity, inaugurating a rush to find a cure, a rush that ultimately helped shift the American medical establishment toward research-based practices. First, a pair of German medical doctors documented the physical existence of the syphilis spirochete in 1905.[19] The following year another German researcher, August von Wassermann, created a reliable diagnostic test. And, perhaps most importantly, in 1909 Paul Ehrlich synthesized Salvarsan (arsphenamine), which rather effectively treated syphilis in its early stages.[20] Salvarsan—or 606, as it was called—was an unstable arsenical compound, a yellow powder that had to be carefully handled in sealed containers prior to being mixed with liquid for injection.[21] These medical discoveries, which sought to both explain and cure syphilis, occurred within the context of shifting, yet still contested, perceptions of insanity itself. Practitioners—some of whom may have previously believed immorality caused madness—increasingly turned to modern laboratory science to understand the origins of insanity.[22] As psychiatrists struggled to validate their work as a legitimate field of medicine, discoveries about syphilis helped establish psychiatry as both important and modern, which ultimately helped elevate its acceptance and prestige.[23] Thus syphilis research purportedly helped not only insane patients, but also the physicians who treated them. Undoubtedly, physicians with advanced training from German universities, which were understood to offer the most modern scientific knowledge, helped usher along some of these transitions. The new understanding of the role of infectious disease as a cause of insanity combined with a growing interest in research ignited the search for new syphilis treatments and hopefully even a cure, what many at the time referred to as the illusory "magic bullet."[24]

Although syphilis only rarely progressed to neurosyphilis, general paresis—as physicians often referred to it—was nonetheless deeply feared because of its complete physical and mental devastation, lack of cure, and near-certain fatality.[25] The resulting symptoms, which included loss of speech and memory, severe dementia, hallucinations, emotional disturbances, physical paralysis, delusions of grandiosity, and eventually death, devastated those unlucky enough to contract the disease. And unlike early-stage syphilis, neurosyphilis failed to respond to treatment with Salvarsan or other arsenicals.[26] This was the context in which Superintendent Bahr sought experimental therapies for use at CSH. As was his habit, Bahr looked to Europe for guidance. He set his sights on what appeared to be the promising work of Wagner-Jauregg.

Julius Wagner-Jauregg's malaria therapy treatment, or "fever therapy" as it was initially known, drew on the nineteenth-century observation that high fevers suffered by people experiencing mental troubles appeared to have a beneficial effect on their mental state.[27] Wagner-Jauregg himself acknowledged that the concept had roots in antiquity, with both Hippocrates and Galen making similar observations.[28] In 1888, after Wagner-Jauregg observed similar effects of fever on patients at the Asylum of Lower Austria in Vienna, he tentatively embarked on experimentation with fever treatment, while worrying about the ethics of inducing fever as a treatment for madness.[29] His initial failed work with streptococci-induced fever caused him to briefly stop the experimentation, before starting up again using tuberculin as the fever inducer.

In 1895 the prospect of treating paretic patients apparently assuaged Wagner-Jauregg's ethical concerns, because he restarted his experimentation in that year, rationalizing the treatment on the grounds that neurosyphilis was incurable.[30] Wagner-Jauregg decided that experimental treatment was worth the risks and the pain for patients suffering from general paresis because they faced the near certainty of death. In 1917, during the First World War, he used malaria as the fever-inducing agent for the first time. These initial treatments started off poorly, as Wagner-Jauregg unintentionally injected his patients with malaria tropica, a lethal strain of malaria that failed to respond to quinine. The deaths of three of the four patients caused Wagner-Jauregg to retreat from his experimentation yet again. But by the 1920s, he was back at it, and Wagner-Jauregg's malaria therapy, which, according to him, resulted in the "cure" of six out of nine patients, became something of a global sensation.[31] In fact, in 1927 Wagner-Jauregg won the Nobel Prize in Physiology or Medicine for his work on the malaria treatment of syphilis. Wagner-Jauregg had been considered by the Nobel Committee as early as 1924, but, as his biographer wrote, "one prize committee member, a Swedish professor of psychiatry, could not be persuaded to recommend the award to a 'physician who injected malaria into a paralytic, because he was in his eyes a criminal.'"[32] This criticism reflected the real tension and uncertainties that existed regarding the malaria treatment. Even as psychiatrists and medical researchers globally (and in the United States) became increasingly enamored with this potential cure for neurosyphilis, concerns about the ethics of this experimental therapy emerged and persisted. Given that in the following decade Wagner-Jauregg began to embrace both eugenics and Nazism—even seeking membership in the Nazi Party—these early concerns seem particularly prescient.[33] Wagner-Jauregg's advocacy of both movements in the years before his 1940 death raises further ethical questions about experimental malaria therapy and its impact on the lives of medically incarcerated women and men.[34] In the 1920s, however, as Wagner-Jauregg was busy winning the Nobel Prize, the excitement over a possible cure seemed to drown out any ethical reservations. Certainly that was true in Indiana, where Superintendent Bahr identified Dr. Bruetsch—Wagner-Jauregg's former student—as the key to the crisis in Indianapolis. Bringing Dr. Bruetsch to CSH ensured the arrival of both malaria therapy and its ethical complexities.

Indianapolis, Indiana

Dr. Bruetsch's arrival in Indiana in the early 1920s occurred during a historical moment of isolationism, intensifying racism, and the melding of previously distinct white ethnic immigrant groups into a dominant white majority.[35] Although the midwestern city of Indianapolis may seem a surprising location for an internationally known experimental medical research project, both the city and its larger midwestern landscape play a starring role in the story of malaria therapy. After all, Bahr and Bruetsch sought not only to identify a cure, but also to situate Indianapolis and CSH more specifically as leaders within a national medical research community. Historians of the Midwest, who have noted a paucity of historical, social, and cultural scholarship on the region, have been working to rectify this academic neglect since at least 2015, with more intentional focus on midwestern urban and rural spaces. Nearly a century before this renewed academic attention on the Midwest as a distinct cultural region, Drs. Bruetsch and Bahr quite possibly felt similarly disregarded in their roles as midwestern physicians and medical researchers.[36] After all it was the coastal and southern urban hospitals that typically built and sustained prominent research centers. And even within the Midwest itself, the cities of Chicago, Minneapolis, and Detroit tended to outshine Indianapolis as important urban centers. Thus, there is a way in which Bruetsch and Bahr's professional desire to make Indianapolis and their CSH research work *known* prefigures the more recent desire on the part of academic historians to *know* the Midwest as a region. Shining a light on the malaria therapy project in Indianapolis both contributes to and reveals the history of Indianapolis as a(n overlooked) midwestern city.

By the 1920s the city of Indianapolis—a region with a rich Indigenous history—had been intentionally shaped into a majority-white city with little connection to its Indigenous past.[37] The persistent contemporary absence of Native history in the popular collective mind reflects a similar process of erasure of Native peoples that occurred over the course of the nineteenth and twentieth centuries, as the state of Indiana solidified its political and social culture. As white migrants moved in, encroaching on Native spaces, an intentional whitening process occurred, which constructed the state itself as "white."[38] After Indiana became a state in 1816, the Miami Tribe—Indigenous to the region—began a decades-long process of negotiation that ultimately resulted in their loss of land and removal. These negotiations culminated in an 1840 "treaty" in which the federal government secured both the 760,000-acre Big Miami Reserve and a promise that the remaining Miami would relocate to Kansas within five years. The Miami attempted to accommodate the growing numbers of Anglo settlers in the mid-nineteenth century, but despite their attempts at compromise, they ultimately lost everything, through both cession of lands and forced removal.[39] Only those Miami who completely assimilated into white society managed to escape removal and exclusion.[40] Thus, by the end of the nineteenth century, despite the continued presence (albeit in smaller numbers) of Indigenous peoples in Indiana, the state had nonetheless become solidly white through the intentional practices of removal and erasure.

Some twenty-five years later, when twenty-seven-year-old Dr. Bruetsch arrived in the capital city of Indiana, he found himself one of a dwindling number of German immigrants in the midwestern state. Although Indiana's late nineteenth- and early twentieth-century immigrant population remained steadfastly small, in 1890 Germans accounted for 77 percent of that foreign-born total.[41] Between 1890 and 1914 German immigration to Indianapolis increased, with German immigrants creating strong and influential networks in the growing city. Indeed, the Indianapolis German community played an important role in shaping Progressive Era arts and music as well as public health. The construction of the Indianapolis City Hospital, which served the city's poor and indigent population, represented the culmination of German efforts, and German-language newspapers thrived even as city schools taught German classes. German churches as well as cultural and social organizations also boomed during this time.[42]

But the coming of the Great War halted not only the flow of German migrants, but also the existing community's influence. Indeed, in the aftermath of World War I, a backlash against all things German resulted in the diminishment of the German language as well as the community's thriving social organizations. As one scholar put it, nationwide, "there were numerous Schmidts who became Smiths and Muellers who became Miller."[43] This renaming experience took place for Indianapolis Germans as well. Thus, by the time Bruetsch arrived during the postwar period, he was a relative rarity, a recent immigrant in a midwestern land inhabited primarily by white, native-born residents, some of whom had eschewed their own German roots and many others of whom had grown leery of foreign-born migrants in the wake of the Great War. But though his immigration status may have marked him as unusual in the mid-1920s, Bruetsch's whiteness placed him quickly within the dominant white majority. And this white majority continued to control the social and political economy of the city in the 1920s, to the intentional exclusion of all others.

The Great Migration, which sent millions of Black southerners north and west in search of jobs and economic, political, and social freedom, occurred alongside rising nativism, xenophobia, and racism in those regions. Although Black migrants to the Midwest helped transform the culture of the region, they found themselves unwelcomed by the majority-white descendants of European immigrants in these midwestern cities.[44] In fact, as one scholar has noted, African American migrants to the Midwest were often perceived by the white majority as "a problem to be diagnosed and treated."[45] Certainly this was the case in Indianapolis, where the nativism and racism that enveloped the nation in the 1920s were in no short supply.[46] Federal immigration restrictions of the 1920s resulted in a significant decrease in the already slow stream of external migration to Indianapolis, further solidifying the white majority. Meanwhile, however, the African American population in the city increased more than 28 percent over the decade, bringing the total number of Black Indianapolis residents to forty-four thousand in 1929.[47]

This increase in the Black population resulted in significant white hostility and racism toward the relatively small African American community. The same impetus toward constructing Indiana as white that had resulted in removal and erasure of Indigenous peoples in the nineteenth century resulted in hostility and backlash against Black migrants in the twentieth century. Meanwhile, Black migrants to Indianapolis and other northern cities found themselves negotiating not only northern racism but also the disappointing reality of their new homes.[48] This was evident in Indianapolis, where racism prompted hospital and housing segregation, which in turn resulted in significant health and welfare disparities for Black residents. Indeed, a 1927 report on race and racism in the health-care system recorded widespread hospital segregation, noting that both the university system of hospitals and most of the religiously affiliated hospitals refused to care for Black patients. In one case, at Saint Vincent Hospital, the mother superior acknowledged that at one time the hospital had taken in "colored patients," but white people had "made such a fuss" that it became unsustainable.[49] Thus, Dr. Bruetsch's arrival in Indianapolis coincided with an explosion in racial hostility toward Black Indiana residents that made its way into every facet of life, including health care. Chapter 4 explores this reality in more detail.

The Malaria Therapy Treatment Begins at CSH

Before there was malaria therapy in Indianapolis, there was malaria. Indeed, some historical irony is embedded in the intentional cultivation of malaria as a therapeutic medical treatment in the city. After all, malaria itself was (and is) a lethal disease, one that prompted significant fear among the white settler population in the early nineteenth century.[50] Throughout the 1820s, as the first white migrants (who numbered just over one thousand by the end of that decade) settled on the land that would become Indianapolis, they began to experience what a historian of St. John the Evangelist Catholic Church noted to be a "strange sickness."[51] The white settlers and physicians referred to malaria, which terrified them, as "'fever and ague,' . . . 'chills and fever,' or sometimes just the 'shakes,'" due to "the violent shaking attendant on the chills, which marked the epidemic." At its worst, the "yearly siege," as it became known, claimed seventy-two lives in one year, nearly 10 percent of the total population at the time.[52] Although the fear of malaria ebbed over the next several decades, such that it no longer posed a particularly potent threat during the Progressive Era, it had nonetheless historically made its presence known and feared in a way that makes clear that the prospect of intentionally injecting someone with malaria must have been freighted.

If nothing else, public memory elicited an awareness that malaria could be lethal, thus the ethical conundrum of injecting one deadly disease to cure another permeated the initial discourse. In 1925, reporting on the earliest malaria injections in the United States, the *New York Times* captured this wariness: "and perhaps only in relation to an ill as hopeless as paresis has been would it be deemed either safe or ethical deliberately to infect a man or woman with a disease that has devastated whole countries and, according to some authorities, has toppled over several civilizations."[53] Back in Indianapolis, Superintendent Bahr perhaps unwittingly acknowledged this concern in his 1925 annual report, which first introduced the malaria therapy experiment to the board of trustees and the Indiana governor. In an effort to provide reassurance that injecting malaria into patients posed no threat to the general Indianapolis community, Bahr wrote, "Since the malarial fever has been endemic in Indiana, we used the utmost precautions and kept the first patients in screened rooms." And even beyond these precautions, Bahr noted that experiments in Vienna, Austria, had recently proven that "inoculation malaria is not transmissible through the bite of the anopheles."[54] Regardless of this latter claim, fears regarding the potential for community transmission persisted throughout the nation at sites where malaria therapy was used. Of note, however, Bahr's concern voiced here centered on the need to prevent malaria in the general community, rather than on any articulated worry about the ethics of injecting the painful and potentially lethal disease into institutionalized women and men.

Whether or not they had ethical concerns, Walter Bruetsch and Max Bahr began their malaria treatment at CSH on August 14, 1925, with an eye toward staking out a cutting-edge research position. In 1929, four years into the study, the pair reported their findings at the American Medical Association annual meeting, held in Portland, Oregon, and by 1930 they had already published widely on their findings over the first five years of the treatment. For Bruetsch and Bahr, the fact of being "first" in the nation, leaders in the deployment of malaria therapy, was particularly important. As Bahr reported to the Indianapolis Medical Society in 1930, "With the exception of one other institution, which soon after introducing this form of treatment discontinued it after a series of experiments, the Central State Hospital was the first hospital in America to apply it continually for a series of years, to observe the clinical outcome in a large number of cases and to note extensively the pathological changes brought about by this line of treatment."[55] By 1930 malaria therapy had become an accepted, even standard treatment at many institutions nationwide, but—at least according to Bahr—Indianapolis's CSH was a research leader in its inception.[56]

Even if Bahr slightly exaggerated his claim (at least two institutions, Saint Elizabeths Hospital in Washington, DC, and Manhattan State Hospital in New York, were one to two years deep into their own malaria experiments by the time CSH began), articulating themselves and their work as front-runners in this pathbreaking treatment clearly meant something important to the two CSH researchers in terms of their professional standing.[57] Bahr claimed that it was the sustained, multiyear nature of CSH's experimental work, accompanied by Bruetsch's expert clinical observation and research notes, that made their work worthy of the designation "first." Importantly, in their efforts to highlight the significant role played by CSH in the wider medical field, Bahr and Bruetsch clearly articulated their position that malaria therapy was not just a *treatment* option, but rather an intentional, sustained *research* project as well. In claiming credit for being the first mental institution in the nation to engage in what they noted to be a long-term research-based endeavor, they also highlighted its experimental nature.

For Bruetsch, the research project became every bit as important as the treatment it offered, and the culture of medical research at the time solidified his role as a leader in the field. Pre–World War II clinical research highlighted cooperative group studies rather than scientifically controlled experimentation, ultimately prioritizing the researcher and their skill as the centerpiece of the research endeavor.[58] This cultural norm of the time—the prioritizing of the individual researcher over methods—contributed to a lack of uniformity in treatment protocols nationwide, even as it also lent a certain authoritative weightiness to physicians' individual beliefs and medical conclusions. Thus, Bruetsch's centrality to the malaria therapy treatment at CSH was supported and nourished by the cultural and historical expectations regarding medical research at the time.

Given this heavy emphasis on the lead researcher, it is perhaps not surprising that even though malaria research programs began springing up throughout the nation in the 1920s, these programs functioned differently at each individual institution engaged in the experimental treatment. Indeed, the variability associated with syphilis treatment more broadly became characteristic of neurosyphilis research as well, demonstrating one way in which research and treatment overlapped.[59] The initial malaria therapy experiments varied so significantly that they became nearly impossible to compare. For instance, Manhattan State Hospital allowed for its patients to have seven to eight "paroxysms" (fever spikes with chills and rigor) before treating them with quinine. Meanwhile, researchers at Saint Elizabeths Hospital permitted patients to spike fourteen to sixteen fevers over the course of several weeks, with some receiving quinine and others left to fight off the malaria on their own. Some Saint Elizabeths patients also received follow-up treatment with Salvarsan, making it challenging to determine whether their outcomes resulted from the malaria or the arsenical.[60] In 1928, seeking to combat these inconsistencies across the nation, the Committee on Research in Syphilis assembled the Cooperative Clinical Group Study—which Dr. Bruetsch would join in 1937—in what ultimately amounted to a failed effort to create a unified syphilis treatment protocol to be used at clinics nationwide.[61]

Dr. Bruetsch and the Malaria Treatment

Although multiple methods of inoculation existed, at CSH doctors transmitted malaria to their patients via blood injection from one malaria patient to another. This was the method first cultivated by Wagner-Jauregg (he opposed the alternative mosquito-cultivated method, which he feared was too dangerous), and it was the method used by Bruetsch as well.[62] But the injection method presented its own dangers. First, worries persisted about the possibility of malarial outbreaks in locations where *Anopheles* mosquitos (mosquitos capable of transmitting malaria) lived at or near the institutions that were providing injections. Although this fear did not appear to materialize in any systemic way, it was much discussed nationwide, and anecdotal reports suggest that medical providers may have contracted malaria on occasion.[63]

A second fear arose from the inherent risks associated with transferring blood-borne pathogens from one patient to another. In the first four years of treatment, CSH managed to use the same single strain of malaria, passing the malaria-infected blood directly from one patient to the next 175 times. Bahr and Bruetsch acquired that initial strain of malaria from a patient at City Hospital; the patient had come down with wild-caught malaria after returning from Arkansas.[64] This initial strain proved so successful that Bruetsch even supplied it to outside physicians over a dozen times, meaning that CSH became a malaria treatment resource for institutions nationwide. And yet, injecting patients with malaria-infected blood carried the potential of spreading diseases beyond just the malaria parasites; on occasion this risk materialized. Bahr and Bruetsch were forced to let that initial successful malaria strain die out after discovering that it had become contaminated with staphylococcal bacteria. "Unfortunately," Bahr admitted, "this patient was used as the donor for the inoculation of several other patients."[65] After discarding the infected strain, CSH acquired its second strain of malaria from the New York State Psychiatric Institute. The ease with which Bruetsch located a new malarial strain suggests that within just four years, malaria treatment had become much more widespread and accepted throughout the nation. Of course, according to Dr. Bruetsch, CSH was instrumental in facilitating this widespread use of malaria therapy. After all, CSH intentionally functioned as an educational hub and supplier of certified malarial strains for the nation.[66]

If all went well during the malaria injection process, Dr. Bruetsch hoped that his patients would spike a series of high fevers over the course of several weeks; once physicians determined that a sufficient number of fevers had been reached, they treated the patients with quinine to cure the malaria. In the first five years at CSH, Bruetsch reported that the treatment cured as many as 30 percent of patients. An additional 40 percent of malaria-treated patients remained hospitalized, and 25 percent worsened and died. Though Drs. Bruetsch and Bahr did not discuss it much, at least 5 percent of patients died during the treatment itself.[67] These statistics did not necessarily take into account spontaneous recoveries or relapses, but Bruetsch's initial cure rate was in line with that of other hospitals engaged in malaria therapy in the 1920s.[68] And yet none of these statistics considered the patients' experiences of treatment, experiences that were undoubtedly grueling and painful.

Bruetsch's self-reporting regularly highlighted the positive aspects of the study, and in fact he seemed able to turn even the least desirable outcomes into useful additions to the research project, with patient deaths becoming opportunities for more knowledge. Researchers sought not only to prove the efficacy of malaria therapy for curing neurosyphilis, but to explain how and why it worked. The most prominent theory rested on the assumption that the high fevers caused by an infectious agent (in this case malaria) ultimately killed the syphilis spirochete that wreaked havoc in the brains of the patients who were afflicted. As several syphilis researchers including Bruetsch noted, in laboratory experiments syphilis spirochetes died at a temperature of 107–10°F, but humans could not survive such high temperatures.[69] If the heat of a fever explained the cure in full, then ostensibly one could replicate high bodily temperatures without an infectious agent; indeed, some researchers explored this idea using various artificial heat chambers, and yet Bruetsch and many other syphilis researchers favored the fevers produced by infectious disease.[70]

Dr. Bruetsch claimed it was more than just the fever that halted disease progression. In a 1928 article published in the *Journal of Nervous and Mental Disease* and coauthored by Bahr, Bruetsch looked to two patients who had died during the malaria therapy to provide pathological evidence of serological improvement, a marker that he viewed as superior to clinical improvement alone. One of the patients, "a man aged 56," was the fiftieth patient to receive this particular malaria strain. The disease progressed normally, with the patient experiencing no symptoms for five days, followed by daily fevers of up to 105°F. Bruetsch noted, "At the height of the seventh paroxysm, which occurred at midnight, the temperature was 104 degrees F. . . . At 12:30am the attendant returned to the bedroom and found the patient dead."[71] Bruetsch found this to be an excellent case study for autopsy, remarking that he was able to glimpse the changes occurring within internal organs during an actual paroxysm. Citing earlier researchers' claims that the dilatation of blood vessels caused by the infectious disease was just as important as the fever, Bruetsch argued that the histopathological changes that occurred in internal organs were integral to the efficacy of the malarial therapy. He claimed that the best results were those seen in patients for whom "a violent reaction of the reticulo-endothelial system" had occurred.[72] Remarkably, then, Bruetsch used the cases of patients who had died during their malaria treatment to prove the efficacy of the treatment itself. For Bruetsch, the microscopic changes he observed in internal organs after death signaled success regardless of the death itself.

As Dr. Bruetsch further developed his malaria claims by studying those who died, he gained significant professional esteem in the process. For instance, Bruetsch used the case of "Mrs. A.M.S., 61 years of age," yet another patient who died during malaria treatment, as a case study to illustrate his claim that malaria itself (not just the fever) successfully altered tissues in such a way as to cure neurosyphilis. Mrs. A.M.S. was admitted to CSH on June 23, 1923, and in 1926 she was injected with malaria, becoming the ninety-seventh patient on the same strain. For nine days she spiked fevers of 104–5°F. On day ten, with the fever hovering at only 100°F, she became restless, and she died the following day. Mrs. A.M.S. spent her final days feverish, chilled, and uncomfortable, possibly scared and anxious. Yet, despite the fact that she succumbed to malaria, Bruetsch turned the patient's death into a research success, not only publishing his findings but also presenting them as the basis for the scientific exhibit *The Malaria Treatment of General Paralysis*, which was shown at a symposium on the malarial treatment at the annual meeting of the German Psychiatric Association, April 9–11, 1931, in Breslau, Germany.[73] In detail, he described his pathology observations of each of her many organs. Mrs. A.M.S. may have died from malaria, but she also became the research data that continued to catapult both Dr. Bruetsch and CSH to international prestige, in many ways underwriting Bruetsch's 1931 journey to Germany. By the time of the demise of malaria therapy in 1949, Bruetsch had firmly established that "elevated temperature is only a minor factor of a number of highly complicated and separate phases which make up the mode of action of malaria therapy."[74] His lasting theory for understanding how and why malaria may have worked to cure neurosyphilis was built on those patients who died as a direct result of the treatment itself.

Throughout the 1930s Dr. Bruetsch continued his experimentation with malaria at CSH, shifting and perfecting his medical conclusions in the process, as he became one of the world's leading experts in the treatment of neurosyphilis. By 1930, some 240 patients had received malaria therapy. By 1934, hospital records note that 400 patients had been treated with malaria, and more than 100 shipments of malarial blood had been sent out to physicians in the region and across the nation.[75] Bruetsch and Bahr continued to highlight the foundational role of CSH in the malaria therapy experiment nationwide, noting the special contributions made by the Indianapolis hospital. Elaborating in the 1930 annual report, Superintendent Bahr wrote,

> In order to demonstrate the therapeutic value of malaria in the treatment of general paralysis, our patients receive malaria only and are not followed up by any other specific treatment. We have carried out this policy in the past five years and feel justified to continue it, particularly since our results compare well with institutions which follow up on the malaria-treated paretic with specific remedies, such as salvarsan and tryparsamide. In this way a most valuable material for clinical and anatomical research has accumulated, which shows clearly that it is the malaria which brings about the negative serology and the clinical improvement.[76]

Bahr's situating of CSH as unique among the nation's public institutions for the purity of its treatment method makes it clear that CSH's approach to patient treatment occurred in tandem with considerations about the professional positioning and prestige of the hospital as an increasingly prominent research institution.

For the first eight years of his research, Bruetsch remained firmly committed to treating patients only with malaria. Wanting to maintain the purity of his research database, he opposed the types of follow-up with additional therapies that were sometimes used at other institutions. Bruetsch touted the purity of his data, noting its increasing usefulness for comparisons with other forms of treatment. His certainty that his positive outcomes could be directly attributed to malaria (as opposed to any other treatment) supported his overall claim that the tissue changes brought about by the malaria were what allowed for a heightened immune response and eventually thwarted the syphilis spirochete. By 1932, however, having firmly established CSH as a national, even international, biomedical research center, Bruetsch began to experiment with different types of follow-up care added to the malaria therapy. For instance, beginning in May 1931, some malaria-treated patients were given Stovarsol, an oral arsenical first introduced in France. A year later, CSH added the popular German practice of requiring patients to sit under ultraviolet lamps following their malaria treatment.[77] By summer 1932, then, CSH patients increasingly followed this new combination protocol, which called for first malaria treatment, followed by a course of Stovarsol by mouth and fifteen sessions of ultraviolet radiation.

Penicillin and the End of Malaria Therapy

When in the early 1940s penicillin became available, Dr. Bruetsch engaged in further experimentation, adding new information to his growing research database, and further cementing both his and CSH's roles as national leaders in neurosyphilis treatment and research. In 1944 the National Research Council requested that Bruetsch begin experimenting with penicillin-only treatment to compare the outcomes with malaria-only treatment. According to Bruetsch, he and CSH were selected because the Indianapolis institution held "the largest case material treated with malaria alone," the result of more than two decades of careful observations.[78] Thus, again according to Bruetsch, CSH was the natural and best choice for comparing outcomes of patients treated with malaria alone and patients treated with penicillin alone. In other words, the National Research Council viewed Bruetsch and his institution as prominent and experienced enough to take on this important experimental project. Bruetsch answered the call, engaging in both experimentation with penicillin-only treatment as requested by the National Research Council, and experimentation with a combined malaria-penicillin treatment, which proved to be Bruetsch's preferred treatment for several years.

Penicillin eventually changed everything, but Bruetsch, who had thrown in his professional lot with malaria, was initially reluctant to embrace this new treatment option. Although the penicillin mold was first discovered by the British medical researcher Alexander Fleming in the 1920s, few researchers advanced this discovery in its first decade. The recognition that penicillin mold contained antibiotic qualities did not become particularly useful until further research began in earnest, in the early 1940s. Researchers Ernst Chain and Howard Florey took the necessary steps to move Fleming's discovery forward.[79] Eventually Florey moved penicillin research to the United States with funding from the Rockefeller Foundation so that the significant challenges posed by mass production could be tackled. As a result, the first commercially produced quantities of penicillin were used in human patients in the United States in 1942 and 1943. A Connecticut woman, Anne Miller, became the first American recipient of penicillin in 1942; although she was reportedly near death with a fever of 107°F, penicillin miraculously saved her life.[80] After World War II, though production challenges continued, the life-saving antibiotic increasingly became more widely available to the public. Ultimately, penicillin—not malaria—became the long-sought-after magic bullet that could cure syphilis.

And yet, before penicillin's triumph, throughout the mid-1940s, Bruetsch remained convinced that malaria therapy played a crucial role in the treatment of syphilis, so much so that he continued to argue in favor of a combined penicillin-malaria treatment many years past the point that such a combination seemed questionable to others. As late as 1946 Bruetsch published his belief in the superiority of this combination treatment in the *Journal of the American Medical Association*. Even upon challenge by other doctors, Bruetsch insisted that the combination was more successful than penicillin alone, and he worried that the latter option could be "hazardous" to patient outcomes.[81] So convinced was he about the superiority of the combination treatment that the death of one patient who received the combination struck him as entirely perplexing. Writing about his surprise (and perhaps distress) in his research notes, Bruetsch recalled that he had hand-selected this forty-three-year-old male patient, whom he considered to be "a good risk," in part because he had been "in fine physical condition." Bruetsch elaborated, "Very shocking experience. Absolutely mystery [sic] as to what caused this disaster."[82] Perhaps it was less the death itself that Bruetsch found shocking, and more the fact that the patient's death contradicted his otherwise confident belief in the combined penicillin-malaria treatment as the syphilitic patient's very best hope.

And yet, despite Bruetsch's initial resistance to the penicillin-only treatment, by 1949 he had changed his tune, admitting that the malaria therapy was not "an ideal mode of treatment." Despite his own preferences, he acknowledged that malaria was being replaced by penicillin. Even so, Bruetsch continued to stand by the efficacy of malaria therapy for the treatment of syphilis-induced madness, noting that while "individuals vary greatly in their defensive powers, and therefore this type of therapy cannot be expected to be curative in all cases," in those whose immune systems were receptive, the malarial fevers could indeed begin a process of physiological change that could lead to "complete cure."[83] Thus, even as Bruetsch recognized and accepted the scientific shift toward penicillin, he nonetheless continued to favor malaria as a potential cure for neurosyphilis. Perhaps after decades of research with more than a thousand patients, it was difficult to let go of his own magic bullet.

Conclusion

In spring 1931—more than a decade before penicillin's triumph over malaria therapy and deep within his research project—Walter L. Bruetsch returned to CSH from his German tour. From both a medical and a professional perspective, the trip had been a success. Bruetsch and Bahr together had widely disseminated their initial conclusions, and in their eyes, the malaria therapy treatment was proving successful. By the time Bruetsch returned, Mabel Smith had been dead for several months. As was the case for so many other medically incarcerated men and women, this "successful" malaria therapy treatment had done nothing to prevent her painful demise from neurosyphilis.

In his 1952 retirement address, Superintendent Max Bahr claimed that the pathology building at CSH represented the first laboratory connected to a "state mental hospital in America." The research conducted in that lab, he noted, "made the institution nationally prominent and added to the medical prestige of Indianapolis." In fact, he concluded, if the work of the pathology lab were "permitted to continue after my retirement, I should consider it the finest memorial to my name."[84] The pathology lab and the research conducted within it did indeed serve as something of a testament to the long medical careers of both Bahr and Bruetsch. That legacy, though, is more complex than perhaps Bahr assumed or hoped at the time. Looking back on his work from the 1950s, Bahr concluded his retirement address by reminding the audience that a "code of ethics" guided medical professionals in their work and motivated them to "comfort the hearts of those upon whom disease and the mist of sadness rests like the fogs upon the mountain peaks, and lift these burdens by our skill and touch of human sympathy."[85] As medical researchers, Bruetsch and Bahr sought to "cure" neurosyphilis first and foremost. And yet even well-intentioned efforts have consequences—some immediately known and others less so—that shape the realities of human experience. The next chapter examines the consequences of the experimental malaria treatment on the individual lives of men and women suffering the debilitating effects of neurosyphilis.

CHAPTER 3

Supplying the Research
Patient Experiences at CSH

Henry Boston, a young farmer, was fine until suddenly he wasn't.[1] Like Mabel Smith, Henry had been young, healthy, and able-bodied prior to the onset of his madness. Henry had been visiting a world's fair when his "psychosis" suddenly began. More than likely Henry attended the 1933–34 Century of Progress Exposition in Chicago, joining the tens of millions of Americans who journeyed to fairs across the country throughout the years of the Depression. Chicago's 1933–34 world's fair, like all the Depression-era fairs, was designed to connect Americans' understandings of themselves as consumers to their hopes for a modern future. The planners designed fairs that highlighted technology and modernism as the economic and social gateways that would lead the nation out of the misery of the Great Depression.[2] In many ways this goal of yoking modernity to progress resembled the hopes of the Indianapolis Central State Hospital (CSH) leaders in the 1920s and 1930s who sought to use the modern malaria therapy treatment to bring about an end to the misery caused by neurosyphilis. Drs. Max Bahr and Walter L. Bruetsch pinned their hopes for a cure—one that would not only save the individual but protect the community—on their new technology. But although Henry's malaria treatment began shortly after his admission to CSH, he became one of the 5 to 15 percent of patients who died as a direct result of the inoculated malaria. Henry's was not the modern future promised by physicians, researchers, and design planners of Depression-era America.

Like Henry, Mabel Smith lost out on her own modern future. Before her malaria inoculation, Mabel was "depressed and irritable" while incarcerated at CSH. Her teeth were in "bad condition," "muscular development poor," "knee jerks completely lost," and "pupil reacts very sluggishly," and she experienced "disturbance of speech," a "staggering gait," and an "almost complete loss of memory for both recent and remote events."[3] Neither her husband, Arthur Smith, nor her parents appear to have communicated much, if at all, with physicians or administrators during her time at CSH. Mabel's patient notes claim no knowledge of her parents' or siblings' health history, suggesting that neither Arthur nor any other family member provided this information. About three months after her arrival at CSH and despite her emaciated state, Mabel was inoculated with malaria. From January 3 through January 21 Mabel lay alone in the medical ward spiking high fevers. By the end of February she died. As with Henry, malaria therapy failed Mabel.

Determined to find a cure for neurosyphilis, Dr. Bruetsch blurred the line between research and treatment in his malaria therapy work. Scholars have noted that such fuzziness is common in the history of medical experimentation.[4] In the muddled space between experiment and therapy, a steady stream of vulnerable and marginalized patients with little hope for survival supplied Bruetsch's syphilis research. Dr. Bruetsch reported that nearly 30 percent of his patients injected with malaria recovered enough to leave the hospital and return to work.[5] In this pre-antibiotic era, malaria therapy looked to many researchers like the illusory magic bullet.[6] And yet, at least 70 percent of patients failed to respond to this treatment. The stories of these patients—those who died—have been largely overlooked, even as their failing physical bodies became increasingly crucial to what was defined as medical progress. Many of these patients had been abandoned at the state hospital by their families. Silenced in both life and death, these stories prove challenging to recover. This chapter argues that inequalities of power, which were embedded in the institutional structure of CSH as well as the predominant medical understandings of neurosyphilis and the evolving concept of informed consent, produced and sustained the biomedical treatment/research at CSH. Rather than being merely an unfortunate consequence of medical progress, these inequalities of power made the experiment possible. Indeed, its success was built on the increasingly disabled minds and bodies of those who suffered, and ultimately died, from neurosyphilis. Reading the files of malaria-treated patients who died against a backdrop of Bruetsch and Bahr's public claims of medical success with malaria therapy reveals a more complex and embodied narrative of this history. This chapter recenters the experiences of women and men who suffered and died from neurosyphilis despite (and in some cases because of) their receiving malaria therapy.[7]

Experiences of Neurosyphilis

Despite the relative rarity of neurosyphilis, its symptoms and consequences were so severe that it was deeply feared.[8] The symptoms of the illness, which included loss of speech and memory, severe dementia, hallucinations, emotional disturbances, physical paralysis, delusions of grandiosity, and eventually death, devastated those unlucky enough to contract the disease. The symptoms could come on suddenly, as occurred with both Mabel Smith and Henry Boston, or they could arrive gradually, slowly stealing a loved one.[9] Although it is difficult to know with certainty how individual women and men experienced the illness, much can be gleaned from medical records and hospital reports, which often described in detail the physical and mental devastation that neurosyphilis caused.

Perhaps one of the most defining features of neurosyphilis was the way that the disease seemed to arbitrarily—and sometimes very suddenly—shift a person from living an able-bodied life to one of acquired disability.[10] For most patients who died, the onset of neurosyphilis changed everything about their experiences of living. Thus, severe physical and mental impairment became a new reality for those suffering from the disease, and in many cases this included profound experiences of pain.[11] Meanwhile, the institutional realities that shaped these women's and men's lives—from family structures to employment to criminal justice systems, and health-care settings—seemed entirely unprepared to accommodate these newly acquired impairments, leaving most to experience disability in lonely and isolating environments, both physically and emotionally.[12] Although Henry Boston had arrived at CSH disoriented, with advanced illness and "grandiose delusions of wealth and power," his hallucinations were mild when compared to those of others who arrived in more significant distress.[13] It is perhaps not surprising that family members often appeared overwhelmed and scared by the onset of symptoms, and that neither families nor City Hospital nor the county jails felt prepared to cope with the extensive impairments wrought by neurosyphilis.[14] In a 1923 letter to staff at CSH, a county jail employee pleaded with CSH to admit a man suffering from untreated general paresis. Although the employee acknowledged that CSH was overcrowded, he also noted that the county jail was entirely unprepared to handle the man's care.[15] This lack of preparedness resulted in an even more pronounced experience of disability.

Intake notes in patient files paint a poignant portrait of the losses experienced by ordinary women and men who developed neurosyphilis and the impacts on their families. Several patients were described as violent and threatening upon admission; some of these threatened suicide while others expressed violence against family and friends.[16] One husband who had his wife committed claimed that she had "threatened me bodily harm," and that she "pounds on dishpans at the hour of midnight, sets out in the yard and screams at midnight." In another case, a man had come home to find his wife with a "roaring fire, the family cat in pan, preparing to roast it." One wife committed her husband after he suddenly began "attacks on his children with a hammer." A boardinghouse owner brought in a roomer who had become "violent and abusive to the family and roomers." A wife who committed her husband recalled that he had begun to "[nail] the windows and doors shut when I leave and won't let anyone in. He is afraid to go out of doors." Yet another woman had "threatened to kill husband and some of the neighbors. Has hidden an ice-pick in bed." And another woman had "made three attempts to set house on fire."[17] Surely such behavior must have been disorienting not only for the individual suffering from neurosyphilis, but for others in the household as well. Family members who witnessed the shame of their child, spouse, sibling, or other relative became susceptible to shame themselves.[18] Highlighting the deep impact of drastically changed and impaired behaviors on family members, one woman lamented that her husband of fourteen years was suddenly and inexplicably experiencing a complete change of personality.[19]

Patients often suffered from hallucinations and what medical providers referred to as "delusions of grandiosity." While some of these hallucinations terrified the women and men experiencing them, others appeared rather benign. Family members recalled that before admission to CSH, one man had suddenly quit his job and "boasted of having a fine farm." Although the gentleman apparently did not have a fine farm, he experienced his delusions with much "good humor." Indeed, he was reported to be "euphoric at all times and never seemed to feel that there was anything the matter with him." In this case and several others, the patients seemed content even if others around them felt alarmed. One woman, for instance, had become suddenly excited one day, and "began to electioneer in loud tone of voice." And in another seemingly benign case, a woman believed that she was a nurse and reportedly enjoyed doing chores around the hospital.[20] Although delusions such as these may not have disturbed the patients experiencing them, they clearly distressed family members and care providers who experienced them as "abnormal," and thus perhaps amplified their own experiences of shame.[21]

Some of the more benign delusions reflected a familiarity with history, politics, and world events, and perhaps even a desire to be helpful, or at least to take some credit for having been helpful. For instance, one man claimed that he "has a deed to the world and will give us all of the gold bonds that we want, and says he raised all of the ships that went down during the war in ten minutes and then went over to Cuba and raised the Maine, took him five minutes to do this." Yet another claimed to have "controlled the Spanish American war and is the person who paid all the bills."[22] In these cases, the "delusions of grandiosity" seem to have been more irritating and embarrassing to those around them than to those experiencing the hallucinations. Although these "mild" or seemingly "benign" hallucinations fundamentally changed a person's life experience, the despair and potential shame regarding this aspect of disability seem to have largely belonged to family and care providers.

Medical staff often recorded hallucinations with irritation or annoyance, regardless of how the delusions affected the individuals experiencing them. Although some hallucinations occurred without disturbing a patient's overall sense of contentment, others appear to have been both terrifying and disorienting, even incapacitating, for those who suffered them. For instance, one patient was noted to be "raving continually except when under sedatives." A distressed woman believed that she "has feet in her bed. Does not want them there. Does not apparently realize that they belong to her." At City Hospital one man had tried to put his bed through the window, and at CSH he became "extremely restless and threatening attempting to strike other patients with chairs."[23] For these patients and others like them, neurosyphilis felt disorienting, overwhelming, and frightening, but their fear does not seem to have prompted any extra empathy or care.

Informed Consent, Physician "Beneficence," and Professionalization

Although the legal concept of informed consent in medical research and experimentation was not codified until 1957, the first two decades of the twentieth century saw multiple legal discussions and decisions that argued in favor of the idea of bodily autonomy for patients. In one such landmark case, in 1914, Judge Benjamin Cardozo determined that "every human being of adult years and sound mind has a right to determine what shall be done with his own body."[24] Even though physicians were not yet required by law to gain the consent of their patients for treatment, there nonetheless existed much discussion among physicians and a growing body of legal decisions regarding ethical practices in medical treatment. Medical historians have identified significant evidence of physicians' concerns for patient consent prior to the legal codification of informed consent.[25] At CSH, although physicians sought family consent for autopsy of deceased patients, they do not appear to have sought consent for malaria therapy treatment, nor for any other specific forms of treatment. This archival absence is notable, given the larger historical context both of the evolving legal and ethical discussions and of the particular history of malaria therapy treatment. Although Judge Cardozo's focus on bodily autonomy for human beings of "sound mind" suggests that insanity complicated the landscape for how physicians thought about who was entitled to patient rights and bodily autonomy, some neurosyphilis researchers nonetheless sought family consent (if not patient consent) for malaria treatment in the 1920s, highlighting both physician awareness of and potential discomfort with the ethical conflict embedded in treating one fatal disease with yet another.[26]

Whether or not Drs. Bruetsch and Bahr participated in these ethical discussions, the field of biomedicine and certainly many of its doctors and researchers were deeply engaged in a struggle over ethical concepts during this interwar era; thus, the doctors at CSH could have been expected to have given thought to the question of patient autonomy in the realms of both experiment and treatment. Medical researchers at Saint Elizabeths Hospital in Washington, DC, sought consent for malaria treatment in the 1920s.[27] And yet, as one scholar has noted, even in places like Saint Elizabeths where written consent was recorded, ethical lapses nonetheless still occurred in clinical practice.[28] At CSH ethical considerations are present in the history of both clinical and research practice. This is largely because at CSH, clinical and research practice overlapped, such that distinguishing between the two becomes difficult if not impossible. As Superintendent Bahr noted in the 1937 annual report, "Both in their regular and research activities the laboratories have become too much a part of the clinical work to be separated."[29] Such entanglements of research and treatment were not uncommon during the interwar era. In her study of experimental radium therapy for cancer patients in the 1930s, for example, Katherine Zwicker notes this same type of overlap, arguing that physicians and scientists working together "blurred the practices of clinical therapy and scientific experimentation." Zwicker further underscores the consequences of such overlap by noting that "patients became objects of study."[30] At CSH, with the boundaries between clinical and research practices similarly collapsed, the distinctions between patient and object also disappeared.

Assumptions about ability and disability lodged themselves squarely within the ethical debates about experimentation and consent at the time. Early twentieth-century medical researchers drew ethical distinctions between healthy subjects and sick patients as well as between therapeutic and nontherapeutic treatments.[31] Medical providers' assumptions about ability and disability affected the moral calculus regarding whether an experimental treatment was considered ethical. Because of their perceived disabilities, institutionalized women and men were not provided the same ethical considerations as their able-bodied peers. Ableism was thus apparent in medical professionals' debates and their assumption that consent would be required for "healthy" persons but not necessarily for "patients."[32] Working hand in hand with this system of power, physician authority and the perceived therapeutic value of the treatment also played a role in determining ethics. If the treating physician reasonably expected the treatment to benefit the patient, then physician "beneficence" stood in for patient consent. Indeed, in such cases, consent was deemed unnecessary. Physician beneficence became the basis on which some medical researchers justified experimental treatment of patients who would otherwise die.[33] Ableist physician assumptions about capacity and productivity shaped both their research and clinical practices.

Given this broader context, it is perhaps not surprising that Dr. Bruetsch and the physicians at CSH do not appear to have sought patient consent for malaria treatment, but their choice is nonetheless meaningful in understanding the connections between disability, consent, and power.³⁴ Bruetsch viewed malaria therapy as a remarkable tool in the effort to cure neurosyphilis. Perhaps he and others believed that their "beneficence" in treating patients with malaria in the hopes of alleviating the symptoms of an incurable and horrific illness provided all the ethical consideration needed. And yet, even though neither the law nor CSH protocol required written consent from these severely ill patients, the records of those who died nonetheless remind us that mentally impaired patients were further harmed by not being given the option to refrain from participating in a painful, exhausting, and potentially fatal treatment.³⁵ Because of their acquired disabilities, CSH patients were assumed to be incapable of making appropriate health choices for themselves. And so, the institution made these choices for them.

Throughout the 1930s, as malaria therapy became more widely accepted, Drs. Bahr and Bruetsch continued to position CSH as an institutional leader in a long-term research and teaching project. Dr. Bruetsch ensured that CSH became both an educational hub that supported the continued research and teaching about neurosyphilis and a

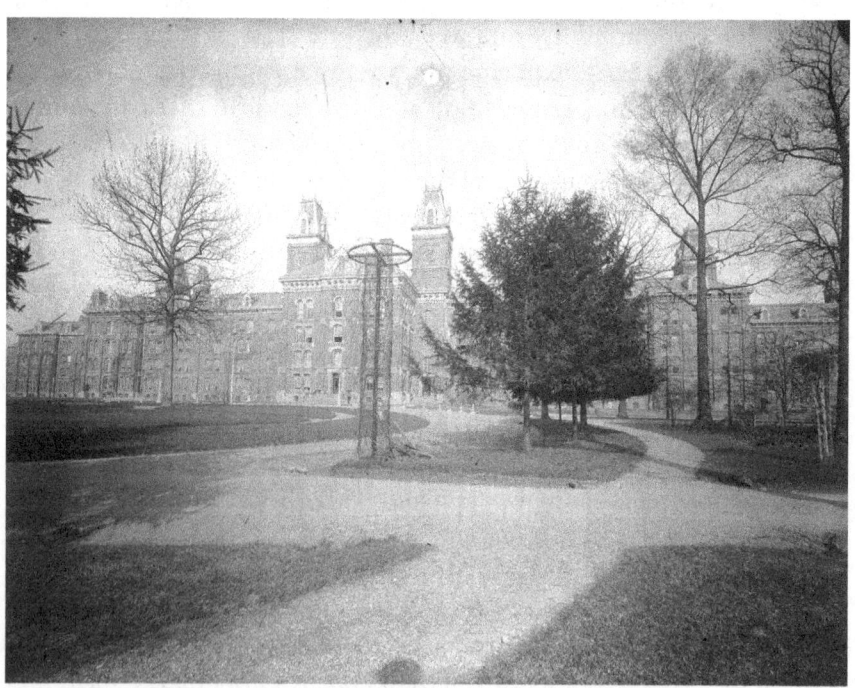

Central State Hospital with Seven Steeples (the women's building). Courtesy of the Indiana Medical History Museum.

supplier of certified malarial strains for the nation.[36] In the 1941 annual report, the board of trustees amplified the importance of CSH's research and educational mission, noting that CSH had by that point become a place "where physicians and students of medicine and law may receive information and instruction which will be of the greatest value and benefit to them and to the community in their practice."[37] Thus, by 1941 Bahr and Bruetsch's efforts had been rewarded; the malaria therapy research project had propelled CSH to national prominence with regard to mental hygiene research, and the hospital had been chosen by the Committee on Research in Syphilis to become an institutional member of the Cooperative Clinical Group Study, whose partners included nationally prominent hospitals such as the Mayo Clinic and Boston Psychopathic Hospital.[38] In addition, in 1944 the National Research Council selected CSH as one of eight sites to conduct coordinated national research into the "malaria therapy plus penicillin combination treatment" for neurosyphilis.[39] But even as CSH and its physicians benefited from the "success" of malaria therapy, and Drs. Bruetsch and Bahr frequently reported on this same success, noting its benefit to the community at large, the surviving records of patients who died tell a more complicated story.

"Carceral Medicine" and Bodily Autonomy

It is difficult to fully grasp the terror that some women and men faced in both their experience of mental and physical impairment and their carceral confinement and treatment at CSH. Highlighting the "political economy of incarceration," scholar Liat Ben-Moshe calls for greater historical recognition of incarceration as a "continuum" and a "multifaceted phenomenon" that encompasses both institutionalization and psychiatrization, in addition to the more commonly discussed criminal justice system.[40] As such Ben-Moshe argues that state mental institutions served a similar carceral function as prisons. Similarly, historian Adria L. Imada employs the term *carceral medicine* to highlight the role of Western medical practices in this continuum of incarceration. As Imada explains, "carceral medicine was a juridical-medical system that incarcerated people and produced knowledge about their bodies."[41] Under Imada's definition, the experimental treatment of women and men suffering from general paresis and the collection and dissemination of the resulting research about their bodies certainly qualify as a form of carceral medicine.

Medical incarceration at CSH meant that women and men suffering from neurosyphilis experienced their sometimes-painful physical and mental impairments alone. As neurosyphilis progressed, the loss of control—including a loss of ability to communicate with medical staff—resulted in frustration and distress for some patients. As recorded in the patient files, one woman "screams and cries continually."[42] Another man "cries easily," and yet another was noted to be "raving continually except when under sedatives." One woman who was noted by staff to be "obscene, violent, and destructive," was also observed to be "nervous, irritable, and extremely emotional. She appears confused and somewhat depressed."[43] The staff presumably found the woman's responses frustrating, but maybe she did not understand what was happening to her, or maybe she was simply in pain. As one scholar of pain has written, "physical pain does not simply resist language but actually destroys it," causing many people in severe pain to lose access to verbal language.[44] Rather than responding with empathy, CSH staff members sought to maintain order, setting up systems to manage patient care that appear to have exacerbated confusion and frustration for many patients. Patients responded in the only ways left available to them: they often cried and thrashed about, chafing against the confusing and controlling measures imposed on them. Although medical staff interpreted this behavior as "difficult" and uncooperative, these expressions of distress and anger can be read from the patients' perspective as completely appropriate reactions to medical incarceration. As one man reported, "I am living in a crazy house. I myself am not crazy."[45] The processes of institutionalization at CSH felt irrational to those who experienced such measures, and their records of distress perhaps demonstrate their best effort at surviving the institution's attempt to exert control over them.

Caring for patients who exhibited symptoms of general paresis proved challenging for staff members, prompting feelings of impatience, irritation, and frustration among staff. The resulting judgmental attitudes are embedded in the patient file notes, as examiners often commented on the "dirty," "untidy," "excitable," and "noisy" nature of their patients with general paresis. Although historian Joel Braslow has argued that the hopefulness brought about by malaria therapy prompted doctors in California to see their general paretic patients as human beings worthy of empathy, I do not see similar evidence of this empathy in the patient records at CSH.[46] More often, physicians and other hospital staff approached malaria therapy not as a source of hope but as just one more in a growing list of potential treatments for neurosyphilis-induced madness, and saw patients in terms of their impairments, not their humanity. For instance, one man who was malaria-treated, released, and later readmitted after relapsing, was referred to by hospital staff simply as "a soiler on B. Ward."[47] If malaria therapy had shifted physicians' perceptions, one might expect that CSH staff would have approached a patient who had previously been "successfully" treated with malaria with more compassion and even optimism for his chances at recovery after readmission. In contrast, staff went so far as to refer to the patient as "a soiler," reducing his complex human situation to the physical impairment that caused him incontinence. The notes go on to describe the patient as "completely demented, disoriented, noisy all the time. Slurring speech."[48] No hopefulness regarding his potential recovery was expressed; instead, his impaired physical and mental state were emphasized without further comment.

Focusing on patient impairments and the potential dangers these posed, physicians and medical staff at CSH frequently resorted to restraining those suffering from general paresis, relying on both physical restraints and sedatives. The practice of restraining patients likely served the institution more than it did patients. The regular and consistent use of restraints to control general paralytic patients who were deemed dangerous or potentially dangerous reinforces the notion of psychiatric care as carceral. As noted in one file, the patient was "always ready to fight and strikes and bites at the attendants as well as the examiner when he is turned in bed. He cries easily. . . . He tears his clothing and bed clothing and has become very destructive requiring a restraint sheet." And another restrained woman was called "vulgar, profane and destructive, tearing up her clothing and bedding . . . no cooperation to medical examination."[49] CSH staff used restraint as a form of physical and social control within the overcrowded and chaotic hospital, frequently referring to patients who needed restraint as "noisy." Such was the case for a restrained woman whom physicians labeled as "extremely noisy" and "extremely untidy," someone lacking any sense of "modesty." Medical staff viewed restraints as medically necessary for dealing with the "convulsive seizures" of neurosyphilis and for protecting patients from hurting themselves and others.[50] Yet such forms of medical control contributed to the carceral nature of hospitalization for people suffering neurosyphilis, an understanding that was only reinforced by news coverage of CSH in the 1920s and 1930s, which consistently referred to patients as "inmates."[51]

Within this context, medical staff who cared for and treated patients participated in the practice of incarcerating disability even as they also faced a tremendous lack of support in their workplace. Superintendent Bahr's annual reports highlighted both the challenging working conditions faced by staff and the lack of high-quality care provided by that same staff. Throughout his tenure, Bahr noted the important role of employees in fulfilling the state hospital's mission, and regularly advocated for their improved compensation. As he began his leadership role in 1924, Bahr noted that the hospital's challenge lay more in *retaining* qualified staff than in *obtaining* staff. This, he wrote, was "due in part to the fact that the hours of duty are long and the association with mental diseases is unattractive to those who are in the least familiar with this class of work."[52] Bahr thus acknowledged both the poor working conditions and the social stigma associated with proximity to madness. One only needed to witness madness in order to share in its shame.

Attending to the needs of the mentally impaired was a highly undesirable and stigmatized form of labor. In 1926 Bahr again highlighted this challenge in his advocacy for improved housing for ward attendants, whose living conditions he described as "unsanitary and deplorable." Noting the way that this poor treatment of employees negatively affected patients, Bahr wrote, "Under the rule of the institution the attendants are compelled to remain constantly at the institution, day and night, with the exception of one-half day each week. This time, both day and night, is spent constantly with their patients; the sleep of the employes [sic] is broken into, their rest disturbed and they take up their duties unrefreshed and unprepared to do justice to the service; it is no wonder that after a short service here they resign to seek other fields more pleasant."[53] CSH had such high employee turnover that during fiscal year 1927, when 281 staff were employed at the hospital, a full 277 of them (98.5 percent) left their jobs. To try to counteract this high turnover, the superintendent advocated for a pension system in addition to improved housing conditions.[54] But the state of Indiana generally did not respond positively to this advocacy, as demonstrated by the fact that Bahr continued to make his case year after year. "Very few people are aware, or even appreciate the detail, work, and duties required of an attendant ... the work is extremely arduous; it is mingled with grave dangers which arise at unexpected moments."[55] Regularly pleading with state government to take seriously the care of those suffering from insanity, Bahr highlighted the difficulties of the work. In doing so, however, he also (perhaps unintentionally) underscored the dangers of being an incarcerated patient at CSH.

Bahr and others knew that the demanding labor required to effectively care for the mentally impaired, combined with the state's completely inadequate funding for compensation, staffing, and facilities, meant that patients at CSH did not receive quality care. The superintendent acknowledged in 1930 that "the highest type of service depends upon a contented mind, a happy disposition, and a well body"—none of which was provided for the medical staff caring for women and men at CSH, as evidenced by his repeated requests for compensation.[56] Bahr's continual efforts to sound the alarm about the threat of poor-quality care provide a glimpse into just how dangerous carceral medicine could be for women and men who found themselves institutionalized. In 1929, for example, Bahr reported the "distressing incident" of two attendants brutally assaulting a patient—Bahr's language suggests that the event was isolated, but the fact that it was recorded at all suggests that additional assaults may have occurred against patients.[57] In 1934 a general paretic patient's family accused hospital staff of having poisoned him. Although the autopsy cited a "ruptured gastric ulcer" as the official cause of death, the family must have had some reason to believe that poisoning may have occurred; there is no further archival information to shed light here.[58] In 1938, after more than a decade of pleas from Bahr, the governor was forced to finally acknowledge the concerns about poor-quality care when Indianapolis newspapers covered the high-profile arrest of a CSH employee whose negligence resulted in the horrific scalding death of a patient.[59]

A persistent problem of overcrowding at CSH created conditions in which patient safety seemed always tenuous. Year after year in asking for funding for facility repair and expansion, Bahr noted the extreme challenge caused by overcrowding. Overcrowding prevented CSH from accepting all patients for whom admission was requested, and it also threatened quality of care for those patients who were admitted. As Bahr repeatedly noted, close quarters hindered proper treatment of the mentally impaired. "The most acute problem that this hospital has to deal with is that of OVERCROWDING," Bahr wrote in his 1926 annual report, emphasizing the last word with all capital letters. "It has greatly interfered with the treatment and the proper classification of the patients." He further reminded the state that this problem had "repeatedly been reported to you but no relief granted."⁶⁰ The overcrowding was so severe that for a period of several months in 1927, at least seventy-two CSH patients were forced to sleep on the floor.⁶¹ Rather than address Bahr's repeated requests for improved and enlarged facilities, the state generally resorted to less expensive temporary measures such as transporting patients to other state institutions when conditions seemed particularly dire.

The problem of overcrowding persisted at the hospital throughout the period of the malaria therapy treatment. Not until the fatal scalding in 1938 did state government officials finally respond more publicly and forcefully to this problem by both acknowledging the abuse caused by negligence and affirming the need for new and expanded facilities, as well as a restructuring of employee care. These were reforms for which Bahr and others had been advocating for decades.⁶² An agonizingly slow process of constructing new buildings and demolishing dangerous structures unfolded, but malaria therapy largely took place amid the chaotic and unmitigated overcrowding.

Although one reason that patients were admitted to CSH, presumably, was to keep them safe, the institution was unable to consistently deliver on this promise; on the contrary, CSH presented a dangerous space for many patients. For instance, several neurosyphilis patients experienced severe radiator burns. A widowed mother of five arrived at CSH feverish and, according to the case notes, just four days later "became violent, found on radiator with hip and feet burnt." The woman's temperature jumped from 103 to 107°F, and she died as a result of the burns. Another patient "burned himself by leaning over the radiator. Large ulcerations developed as the result of this accident."⁶³ In addition to these deadly accidents, a significant number of women and men suffering from neurosyphilis died because of bed sores or ulcers that developed due to their bedridden—and, in some cases, restrained—conditions.

One way that mentally impaired patients resisted medical incarceration was to leave. Each year a number of women and men ran away from CSH. Between 1924 and 1932, the annual reports recorded between fifteen and fifty such "escapes" annually. Many of these women and men had been granted unsupervised "grounds" privileges and simply left the premises.⁶⁴ Their decision to leave as well as the naming of their leaving as "escapes" further reveal patient experiences at CSH to be a point on the carceral continuum.⁶⁵ At least one woman who escaped and tragically died was not accounted for as such by the hospital. Referring to her as an "escaped Central State Hospital inmate," the local press reported that the woman's body was found "in a small closet in a vacant house" on Halloween 1929.[66] Apparently, after running away from CSH, the woman found the abandoned house and sought shelter. Although officials initially thought that the woman had been murdered, an autopsy found that she had not eaten for several days, and that she likely died of either exposure or heart disease. CSH made no mention of the tragedy in its annual report. Notably, it does not appear that many general paresis patients "escaped." The reasons for this are both uncertain and complex. It could be that most of those suffering from general paresis were too incapacitated by their illnesses to attempt escape. Or, perhaps just as likely, those same women and men may have been too closely supervised, restrained, and detained to have had the opportunity to run away, with grounds privileges only rarely granted. Both scenarios may have existed simultaneously. It is also possible that CSH failed to accurately record all escapes, mislabeling some as "discharged" patients and ignoring others.[67]

In addition to running away, women and men expressed their dismay at being incarcerated at CSH through tears and anger. Edith Sutton was devasted when she was readmitted to CSH for a third time.[68] Edith supposedly suffered from "Manic-Depression," but her Wassermann test was positive for syphilis. Despite this finding, she was not treated with malaria, and in fact does not appear to have been treated in any way for neurosyphilis. Because she had previously been twice admitted to and "successfully" discharged from CSH, doctors presumably assumed that her third admission would similarly result in recovery. And yet Edith was distraught upon her return to CSH. Edith cried all the time, "moaning and wringing her hands," begging to go home and worrying aloud that she would never be allowed to leave.[69] With her third bout of insanity, Edith's knowledge about what to expect at the hospital terrified her. Because her peculiar behavior began abruptly, because her Wassermann test was positive for syphilis, and because ten years after her death, her widowed husband succumbed to neurosyphilis at CSH, it seems probable that Edith, too, suffered from neurosyphilis during her third admission to CSH, even though doctors neither diagnosed nor treated her for it. Having previously experienced medical incarceration at CSH, Edith knew even in her mentally deteriorated state that she could not bear another stay at the hospital, and so she fled.

On occasion, women and men activated bodily autonomy by refusing medicine at CSH. For instance, a husband and wife who both suffered from general paresis refused sedatives on the basis of their Christian Science religious beliefs.[70] Recent historical work has found such refusal relatively common among institutionalized women and men.[71] And yet, only a few such cases are recorded in the CSH neurosyphilis files. As with "escapes" this absence may be due to both the significant mental incapacitation experienced by those suffering from neurosyphilis and the high levels of restraint and supervision to which they were generally subjected.

Although resistance may have been challenging for most people suffering from neurosyphilis at CSH, family efforts to assert agency even within the confines of their loved ones' medical incarceration are evident in a small number of archival records. Though families generally seem to have been rather cut off from communication with hospital staff, family-led advocacy (if infrequent) occurred in two primary capacities: pleading *for* malaria therapy treatment and requesting information about a loved one's health status. The first situation arose in a handful of cases in which Drs. Bruetsch or Bahr noted that a patient who was not considered the best candidate for malaria treatment was treated nonetheless, at the insistence of family members.[72] Interestingly, this situation suggests both that there was some space for individual patient advocacy (assuming that one had family members with the time, knowledge, and resources to communicate with CSH doctors) and that malaria therapy eventually became a sought-after, even desirable treatment, at least for some people, despite its experimental status.[73] Malaria treatment was considered cutting-edge therapy, and as such some individuals and families advocated for its administration to their loved ones.

The infrequent family communications with CSH staff that occurred and were preserved offer hints at the ways that some family members struggled to stay connected to their loved one and to resist the totality of medical incarceration. For the most part, CSH medical staff and administrators did not anticipate much if any family intervention in either patients' treatments or their deaths. Outside of autopsy request forms (which are discussed in more detail in chapter 5), CSH staff generally expected that families understood that care and treatment at CSH were facilitated by "experts" who knew what was best for their patients. And for the most part, families did not question these assumptions.

But outliers exist in the archives, as extensive correspondence on the part of the wife of one patient makes clear. Over the course of a four-month period, this woman wrote several letters to Superintendent Bahr, pleading with him for information about her husband and his condition. In her letters she repeatedly asked Bahr to allow her husband to write to her. "I want to know why he don't write to me, and he says he does not get my letters. Dr. Bahr I know you are a busy man but I have such a hard time getting a little money for stamps and I would like when I write to him to have him get my mail." In desperation she even included stamps so that his letters might be properly postmarked. Occasionally, short typed replies from CSH staff answered her increasingly urgent requests. One such response stated, "On checking the records... we find that the customary autopsy blank has never been signed. We ask that you sign it and return at once so that we can complete his record." This was followed by a handwritten note from CSH staff, alerting her that her husband's "condition is regarded as serious and he may not recover from his present acute illness." The wife's final letter again requested information, but this time in the aftermath of death. "I would like to know what you found when you performed an autopsy on my husband's body." And yet, despite the persistent lack of communication from CSH, the patient's wife still closed her letter in gratitude: "thank you very much for your kindness and care to him while there at the hospital."[74] Perhaps CHS staff members failed to fully communicate with families in part because they did not have to. In the cultural power dynamics at work, families understood that they held little recourse in their relationships with a large state institution staffed by medical experts.

Although the wife's expression of gratitude is notable, the impossible conditions under which it was proffered mean that her gratitude may have been the only means available for asserting her emotional autonomy. Perhaps, having experienced the devastating effects of trying to care for a loved one who was suffering from neurosyphilis, some family members did feel relief or appreciation that the hospital stepped in and took over. And yet, even expressions of gratitude took place within a context of unequal power dynamics, wherein desperate families recognized CSH as their last and only hope for dealing with neurosyphilis.

Experimentation and Evolving Criteria for Malaria Therapy Treatment

Patient files are replete with stories of a family history of syphilis, suggesting that the destruction caused by neurosyphilis spared neither spouses nor children (who could contract the disease congenitally). In multiple cases, husband and wife died from general paresis at CSH, and evidence of congenital syphilis is present in many files.[75] Unsurprisingly, physicians linked this real history of congenital syphilis with ideas of "hereditarianism," which undergirded eugenics at the time. Even though there was nothing actually "hereditary" about neurosyphilis, concern about the possibility of passing the infection to children mirrored progressive reformers' fears about hereditary "feeblemindedness" and "degeneracy."[76] As such, malaria therapy can be viewed as a radical intervention and an alternative to other eugenics-inspired "solutions" to what was perceived as the problem of the "unfit." Young patients in particular drove these fears of congenital syphilis. For example, one eighteen-year-old male patient first showed symptoms at age fifteen, when he began to be violent and tried to kill members of his family. His father was also a "paretic," and his grandfather was noted as "insane." In addition, he had a younger sister who was experiencing similar symptoms. The doctor who admitted him determined the cause of his illness to be congenital syphilis.[77] Many other patient records include extensive family histories of general paresis as well.[78] But if malaria therapy promised a potential end to this type of family devastation, the decisions about how it was used and for whom seem to have been somewhat arbitrary.

Although Drs. Bruetsch and Bahr developed an informal set of criteria for determining who would and would not be treated with malaria, these criteria evolved somewhat haphazardly alongside the experiment itself, resulting in inconsistent and rather loosely followed principles of treatment. In one of the first annual reports that summarized the malaria therapy experiment, Dr. Bahr noted that patients were selected and treated with malaria "more or less indiscriminately."[79] That said, Bruetsch and Bahr also acknowledged early on that those who had suffered for a shorter duration of time were more likely to benefit from the malaria treatment, and they identified a number of conditions that contraindicated malaria therapy treatment, such as heart and kidney disease. Nonetheless, these determinations did not necessarily keep the team from administering malaria to patients who had been sick for long periods of time or who suffered from physical contraindications. As Bahr put it, "there is no necessity to adhere rigidly to [treatment criteria], because in the event of the appearance of alarming complications during the febrile attack," quinine could always be administered.[80]

Even as Drs. Bahr and Bruetsch produced additional medical knowledge about malaria therapy, this knowledge was built on the increasingly disabled bodies of those who died. As Bahr wrote in 1927, "It can not be denied that this form of treatment is attended with definite risk for the patient. With a better knowledge of the complications that arise during the rigors, death due to therapeutic malaria will be reduced."[81] Thus, although they preferred to focus on the "successes" of malaria therapy, Bahr and Bruetsch not only recognized its risks to patients but also determined that the production of "better knowledge" was worthwhile and would ultimately reduce those risks. In 1929 the duo even more directly acknowledged this trade-off, writing, "Malaria treatment as any other method of treatment, if applied with insufficient knowledge, endangers the life of the patient." Noting that the risk of mortality had fallen from 15 percent to 2 percent among patients treated, they effectively acknowledged that the earlier deaths had produced the medical knowledge that helped reduce the risk of death.[82]

Despite this awareness, the new and "better" medical knowledge that was produced by the malaria therapy treatment does not appear to have been consistently applied. Rather, inclusion in the treatment protocol was seemingly dependent on Dr. Bruetsch's assessment of who may or may not make a good candidate for the treatment. In several cases, patients who had been living at CSH with syphilis for more than a decade were not treated with malaria even once it became available.[83] One newly arrived woman in the 1930s was treated with "arsphenamine [Salvarsan] only," despite the fact that malaria was certainly available. The woman arrived already feverish, and she quickly declined. Yet even though she was not treated with malaria, Dr. Bruetsch claimed in her autopsy report to have learned something new about malaria, suggesting that "malaria therapy is now even more highly valued because it will prevent a possible increase of plasma cells."[84] In yet another case, malaria therapy was withheld in 1925 because the patient had tested positive for typhoid fever. This patient and nine others were observed rather than treated with malaria; as noted by Dr. Morris, "the intention [was] to observe what a natural disease, such as typhoid fever will do to general paralysis."[85] The medical experimentation at CSH thus extended to withholding treatment. Ironically, Dr. Bruetsch did not agree with the scientific speculation that high temperature alone was responsible for the cure of neurosyphilis. Indeed, much of his own research was intended to demonstrate the incorrectness of this thinking, showing instead the specific mechanism of malaria that was necessary for healing neurosyphilis.[86] Thus, at least in this case, CSH made decisions to withhold treatment not necessarily because it was in the best interest of the patients, but rather because it might produce more medical knowledge.

In other cases, Bruetsch's postmortem notes acknowledge that some patients were treated with malaria who should not have been. In one such case, Bruetsch noted that a patient who died "should not have been inoculated with malaria" due to his poor heart condition.[87] Case notes such as these reinforce the idea that physical health only loosely served as a criterion for inclusion in the experimental treatment. In yet another example, a patient who died as a result of "therapeutic malaria" was noted to have been "a poor risk for malaria since his case appeared to be far advanced."[88] And yet, patients who were deemed "poor risk" due to contraindications were nonetheless inoculated with malaria. In a similar vein, in 1928, CSH decided to give malaria therapy to nine patients who were not suffering from general paresis but rather exhibited symptoms of schizophrenia.[89] The choice to treat these patients seems to have been both experimental and arbitrary.

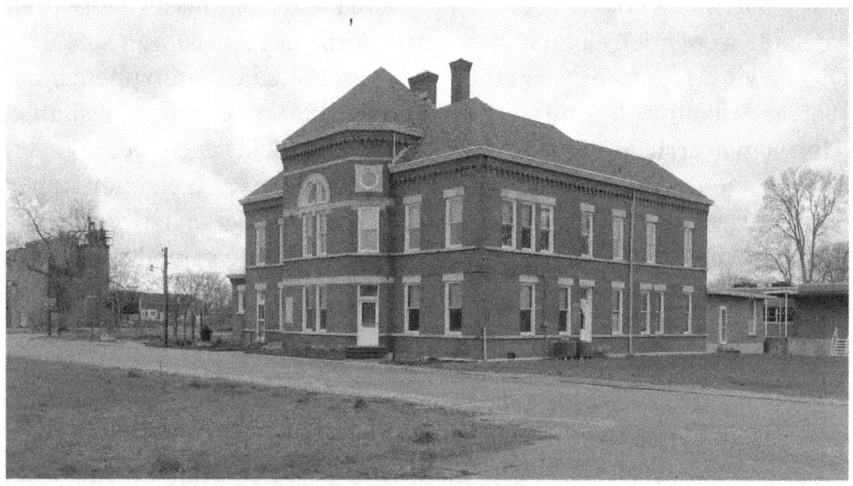

Old pathology building of Central State Hospital, which now houses the Indiana Medical History Museum. Photograph by Christin L. Hancock, 2017.

As a final note on the inconsistent and sometimes dangerous application of treatment criteria, one patient was given malaria just "to keep the strain going." This woman had received malaria treatment upon her initial admission to CSH and showed "great improvement" within months. This initial improvement, however, was followed by a rapid downward turn, with Bruetsch's notes on this patient concluding, "Malaria-treated. Worse." Despite her previously failed malaria treatment, CSH medical staff knowingly inoculated this same woman six years later for no other reason than "to keep the strain going." As a result, she developed a high fever and weakened heart, which caused her death.[90] The woman, who had not benefited in any sustainable way from malaria treatment, was nonetheless treated a second time, and she died as a direct result of that inoculation, despite doctors' efforts to revive her with quinine.

Patient Deaths: Concluding Notes

Although it was Dr. Bruetsch's focus on the malaria therapy "successes" that catapulted the hospital to national and even international prominence as a research laboratory, that professional standing was built at least as much on the 70 percent of patients who did not recover in any meaningful way. Forty percent of malaria-treated patients showed no change or improvement and remained hospitalized, and 25 percent worsened and died (with between 5 and 15 percent dying because of the treatment).[91] It seems that the majority of patients treated with malaria found it completely unhelpful and, in a minority of cases, even lethal. In her history of neurosyphilis and its treatments in Scotland, historian Gayle Davis concluded, "The evidence would suggest that the vast majority of the few patients who were recorded as recovered had in fact received no treatment whatsoever during their asylum stay." Indeed Davis even found that "the majority of those patients who did receive treatment died."[92] Specific numbers are not available for determining similar outcomes at CSH, but it seems clear that even as physicians and researchers like Dr. Bruetsch trumpeted the success of malaria therapy, the actual record can be read in several, sometimes contradictory, ways.

Although Dr. Bruetsch's published work tended not to focus on the deaths associated with malaria therapy, patient files and annual reports reveal that many who died did so during or soon after malaria treatment.

In one such example, Dr. Bruetsch acknowledged that "malaria treatment is considered an absolute failure in this case."[93] For some patients—like the woman who was inoculated just to keep the strain alive—malaria therapy provoked an immediate downward spiral resulting in death. Such was the case for a middle-aged man who died from the malaria. According to Bruetsch's notes, this patient's condition declined precipitously as a direct result of the treatment: "Immediately after patient was inoculated, he stopped eating. . . . The tongue was dry, and the patient could hardly talk. After several days he could not swallow at all, and it became practically impossible to feed the patient. Intravenous glucose was given. He was in a semi-stuporous condition and did not talk to relatives who visited him."[94] Crucially, this patient did receive visitors at CSH, and yet throughout those last few weeks of his life, malaria therapy resulted in his inability to communicate with them. In yet another example of malaria-caused death, the routine administration of quinine (which was supposed to halt the malaria after nine days of illness) failed to stop the man's fevers, which continued to spike up to 102°F for nearly two more weeks. By the time the fevers finally stopped, the malaria had fatally weakened the man's heart, and he died within a few weeks. Yet another patient was treated with a lengthy course of malaria that resulted in nineteen paroxysms, only to die unexpectedly about four weeks after quinine was administered. As Bruetsch recorded, "he called for help, sank to the floor, and immediately died. He had eaten a hearty meal and had laughed and was jolly as usual."[95] Although Bruetsch wondered aloud in his pathology notes what had caused the "patient to die suddenly on the dinner table?" no clear answers were forthcoming. Despite Superintendent Bahr's repeated claims that there was no need to hesitate in treating patients with malaria because the fevers could always be "promptly arrested by the administration of quinine," patient records suggest otherwise.[96] Quinine did not save every patient from death, and researchers who focused exclusively on quinine's efficacy not only failed to account for this reality, but also failed to see patients' experiences of pain as meaningful.

Bruetsch's questioning of the death of yet another patient reveals his own confusion and uncertainty regarding why some patients died from the inoculation. This patient's malaria treatment ended with her sudden death, just eleven days after it had begun. "Why did this patient succumb to malaria," asked Bruetsch before continuing: "No obvious cause was found at autopsy with the exception of the dehydration." Another woman whom Bruetsch had believed to be a good candidate died the day after her last day of malaria treatment. And in still another death due to malaria, Bruetsch suggested that perhaps the patient's inoculation with malaria had not really "taken," as he felt that her "temperature chart was very irregular and never typical."[97] Despite his convictions about malaria therapy, Bruetsch's notes reveal both curiosity and confusion over why some patients died from the treatment. Just as outcomes for treated and untreated patients in Scotland tended to be arbitrary, no clear patterns emerged for Bruetsch at the time of his research regarding why some patients at CSH succumbed to the malaria.[98]

In addition to this confusion, there is also uncertainty regarding the actual number of cases that Bruetsch deemed "successes." For instance, Bruetsch's numbers likely failed to account for spontaneous remissions. Even before malaria therapy began, a well-established characteristic of neurosyphilis was that unexplained spontaneous remissions occurred fairly regularly. These mysterious recoveries were never fully understood by researchers or practitioners. And yet their documented existence made it difficult to draw any firm conclusions about the efficacy of various treatments, including malaria therapy.[99] In addition, some patients whom Bruetsch initially noted as having been cured suffered relapses years later and ultimately died. For instance, one patient who was considered successfully improved from malaria treatment in 1928 and later furloughed ended up back at City Hospital after suffering what was believed to be a stroke; he was readmitted to CSH in "deplorable condition," and ultimately died.[100] Recognizing the possibility for relapse, Bruetsch took care not to classify patients as cured until at least five years after discharge, but even so, some patients were readmitted more than five years after their "successful" recoveries. This reality of the recurrence of disease made any assessment of "cure" rather challenging and ultimately arbitrary, representing just a snapshot assessment of "ability" and health at a particular moment of time.

For women and men at CSH who suffered from neurosyphilis, malaria treatment shaped their experiences of institutionalization and carceral medicine. For those who died, physician "beneficence" was not enough to protect them or positively alter the trajectory of their illnesses. Rather, their increasingly disabled minds and bodies became the research on which the medical knowledge about neurosyphilis and malaria therapy was produced. In the process, malaria therapy solidified inequalities of power and contributed to the construction of disability as nonnormative and in need of medical cure, regardless of how dangerous or painful that "cure" might have been. The next chapter further examines these connections by highlighting the ways that racial and gender ideologies intertwined with constructions of disability to both construct and reflect perceptions of "normal."

CHAPTER 4

Race, Gender, and Neurosyphilis

In many ways Mabel Smith's story of institutionalization and experimental health treatment is not unique. Like nearly one thousand other women and men who were committed to Central State Hospital (CSH) with neurosyphilis during the interwar period, she was inoculated with malaria, and, like many of those other patients, she died. But that is not the whole story. Mabel Smith—and every other person treated at CSH—had an individual life story prior to her institutionalization that marked her as a distinct person. Although as a group the malaria-treated individuals at CSH can be largely classified as "marginalized" (after all, many of them had been abandoned at the hospital, others arrived from poor and working-class families, and all of them suffered mental and physical impairments caused by a venereal disease that marked them as shameful), their individual identities were diverse. Because the malaria therapy included both men and women, Black and white, reflections of gendered and racialized ideologies of the time are evident both in the patient files and in certain medical conclusions made by CSH staff. As a young woman among a group of patients who were predominantly male, Mabel Smith challenges the medical and public health narrative of the time, which focused almost entirely on white men as the victims of neurosyphilis. But Mabel was also a *white* woman, and so her story reveals only one dimension of women's experiences at CSH; her whiteness should be considered within the larger historical context of race and racism, both in Indianapolis and in the national medical discourse. Although Mabel's whiteness did not protect her from institutional power—institutionalization rendered her disabled, abnormal, and unfit for society—the practices employed by medical incarceration nonetheless reinforced social constructions of race, racism, and gender, even within this group already targeted as defective.

Dr. Walter L. Bruetsch's inclusion of Black and white women as well as Black men in his experimental treatment protocol reveals one way psychiatric institutionalization and treatment both reflected and reinforced gender and race ideologies.[1] For instance, at CSH Dr. Bruetsch made medical conclusions based on predominant but erroneous assumptions about biological racial difference, ultimately adding to the medical racism that underscored beliefs about neurosyphilis.[2] In addition, Dr. Bruetsch's and Superintendent Max Bahr's definition of successful treatment relied on gendered notions of productive labor. "Successful" malaria therapy treatment resulted, at least in part, in the return of women to gendered domestic duties in the home. As such, malaria therapy could also be seen as offering the hopeful possibility of a return to "normative" (re)production. When it functioned "successfully," malaria therapy offered a potential cure not just for neurosyphilis, but also for "degeneracy" and its accompanying shame. Yet when it failed (as it often did), those women and men who died or who failed to improve continued to be marked as unfit. Playing a multifaceted role within the political landscape of eugenics, malaria therapy substantiated eugenic thinking with regard to medical racism and gendered assumptions about domesticity, even as its potential success challenged the concept of hereditarianism embedded in eugenics.

The construction of both sets of knowledge—conclusions about racialized medicine and gendered definitions of successful treatment—unfolded within the historical context of a growing medical and social reform embrace of eugenics. In the early twentieth century, eugenic thinking embedded racism in science.[3] The incorporation of racialized medical conclusions based on modern malaria therapy treatment helped solidify the scientific basis for racism, even though it did so within a local context.[4] Malaria therapy treatment of patients of color and women at CSH during the 1920s and 1930s engages all these realities, suggesting the ways that doctors at CSH contributed to larger national and international medical discussions even as this practice played out within the distinctly regional context of the state of Indiana.

Neurosyphilis, Medical Racism, and Malaria Therapy

Like their white counterparts, Black patients at CSH supplied the research for the long-term study of malaria therapy. At roughly the same time that CSH was treating Black neurosyphilis patients, the US Public Health Service—operating some six hundred miles south of Indianapolis in Tuskegee, Alabama—began its infamous experimental *non*treatment of hundreds of unsuspecting Black men suffering from syphilis.[5] For nearly forty years these patients were followed and observed but denied treatment, even after penicillin had been firmly established as an effective and efficient cure. Although the individual experiences of Black patients at CSH and Tuskegee's John A. Andrew Memorial Hospital clearly differed—most obviously with regard to whether they received treatment—institutional systems of health and medicine nonetheless experimented on them all, observing and recording their illnesses as well as their physical bodies in an effort to produce medical knowledge. In both cases medical experts made determinations about medical treatment and research without input from the people most directly affected. Patients in both locations were viewed and processed through similar racially coded lenses, which ultimately produced racialized medical knowledge. Considering the story of malaria therapy through the lens of race further reveals power inequities embedded in medical incarceration.

For most of the early twentieth century, a belief in biologically based differences between racial groups predominated, providing the foundation for racist assumptions in science and medicine as well as eugenic thought and policies. This biological determinism was not new; to the contrary, evidence of it can be found throughout colonial history as well as in eighteenth- and nineteenth-century US histories of medicine and science.[6] Scientific racism underlay southern antebellum proslavery arguments and, after the Civil War, resulted in a medical focus on health disparities for Black Americans that was again biologically based (as opposed to focusing on socioeconomic factors like poverty, the denial of political rights, and white hostility and violence toward newly freed Black Americans). Venereal disease became a special interest of health experts, medical writers, and sociologists, who linked race, infection, and "degeneracy," worrying in particular about the potential threat of contagion to the survival of white America. From the late nineteenth century through the first three decades of the twentieth century, much of the increasing white medical interest in Black American health and illness was predicated on this fear.[7] Leading medical researchers of the early twentieth century relied on eugenic theories about race and inheritance to resurrect and sustain nineteenth-century beliefs about biologically based racial difference.[8] In effect they used the authority of modern science, which was steeped in eugenics, to advocate for understanding disease processes differently on the basis of race.[9] By the 1920s, as the malaria therapy experiment first began in the United States, biological determinism had been long embedded in American legal and medical systems. Meanwhile, the increasingly widespread medical commitment to eugenics—not just nationally, but internationally—created the context in which medical researchers learned, observed, thought, and generated knowledge about syphilis, neurosyphilis, malaria therapy, and race.

Although white men made up the majority of neurosyphilis patients at CSH, Black men and women nonetheless also suffered from neurosyphilis; their presence in the patient files challenges conventional medical beliefs about race and neurosyphilis at the time. Early twentieth-century medical researchers reported racial differences in syphilis, noting higher rates among Black Americans than their white peers; these researchers blamed the disparity on alleged weaknesses and failures of Black populations, a belief that both reflected and underscored deeply entrenched assumptions about white superiority. Ironically, however, these medical observers simultaneously noted lower rates of *neurosyphilis* among Black patients than white patients.[10] White medical researchers claimed that this inconsistency resulted from the fact that more "primitive" brains resisted nervous system disorders; in other words, white doctors alleged that Black cognitive inferiority protected Black men and women from developing neurosyphilis.[11] This persistent belief "that insanity was a disease of 'civilization,'" with peoples deemed "primitive" generally protected from it, shaped much of the American medical understanding of Black madness in the late nineteenth and early twentieth centuries.[12] Meanwhile, Black patients continued to suffer from neurosyphilis, showing up in the admission books of mental institutions from Saint Elizabeths to Tuskegee, and CSH.[13]

Race and Racism in Indianapolis in the Early Twentieth Century

Like their white counterparts, Black men and women who were admitted to CSH in the 1920s and 1930s entered a system of medical incarceration that marked their lives and bodies as abnormal and unfit for the outside world. Unlike their white counterparts, however, Black patients also had to navigate a health-care system that replicated and contributed to the racism of the world outside. Black patients entered a state mental institution that was deeply enmeshed in both an international system of modern medical research and the particular local context of the capital city of a midwestern state. In both contexts, deeply biased assumptions about race and biology profoundly affected Black patients' experiences.[14] Race and anxieties about racial difference shaped the ways doctors at CSH engaged, treated, and observed patients, as well as made medical conclusions regarding malaria therapy and neurosyphilis.[15] The malaria treatment of Black men and women suffering from neurosyphilis at CSH provides a glimpse into the cultural values associated with race in Indianapolis in the 1920s and 1930s, in addition to those that permeated national medical discussions about both madness and venereal disease. These values and assumptions shaped the ways that doctors—who were predominately white—perceived patients, their experiences of illness, and their responses to treatment.

An insular and conservative midwestern city, Indianapolis responded to the growth of its African American population by, among other things, racially segregating its hospitals and health-care facilities. Even as the Black population of Indianapolis increased by more than 28 percent over the course of the 1920s, few of these residents could adequately acquire hospital health care.[16] White hostility resulted in most hospitals within the city refusing to accept Black patients.[17] Moreover, at least 5 percent of physicians in Indianapolis were dues-paying members of the Ku Klux Klan.[18] The Klan of the 1920s gained significant and widespread support in northern states; its commitment to white supremacy was supported by large numbers of Americans, well beyond its actual membership.[19] This pervasive racism, reflected in both racial segregation and the thriving Klan, undergirded all social, economic, and political aspects of life in the city, including its health-care systems.

Racial segregation and exclusion within the medical system in Indianapolis were endemic. A 1927 report on hospital conditions, conducted at the behest of the Indianapolis Foundation, noted the urgent need for hospital beds for the Black community. Only City Hospital, serving the poor and indigent, accepted Black patients, with adult patients racially segregated. This underresourced public facility provided only 42 female beds and 24 male beds for an African American community in urgent need of at least 190 hospital beds. According to the Indianapolis Foundation study, most Black residents intensely disliked City Hospital (perhaps in part because of this system of racial segregation) and "would only go there in dire need."[20] Indeed, the foundation report recommended the construction of a separate "colored" hospital staffed by Black physicians, with a nurse training program for Black nurses. White hostility toward the growing Black community in Indianapolis was so pronounced that leading African American physicians also favored the creation of a separate hospital system for Black residents, even if their reasoning surely differed from that of white leaders like the medical school dean who insisted that "colored and white could not be mixed without creating discord and even open rebellion."[21] These multifaceted efforts to exclude, segregate, and create separate facilities of care for Black residents reflected citywide values and practices of racism, in addition to the Black community's attempts to survive within this unequal culture.

It was within this context of racial hostility and public pressure toward segregation that CSH—as well as the underfunded City Hospital—admitted and treated Black patients.[22] And it was also within this context that Dr. Bruetsch included Black neurosyphilis patients in the malaria therapy research project, apparently perceiving Black women and men to be as valuable—at least in terms of scientific data—as white men. And yet their inclusion did not represent any type of forward racial thinking. On the contrary, the same racial assumptions and racist stereotypes that pervaded society at large are evident in the physician intake notes of Black patients at CSH. Embedded in the detailed life histories are gendered and racialized biases on the part of physicians, who described their Black patients as "filthy, obscene," and "dull and stupid." Stereotypes abound in patient descriptions, with one man judged to be an "emaciated negro of a low type mentality," and another deemed to make an "average living for a negro." Further, a "delusional" Black male patient who suffered from ideas of "grandiosity" was said to be so in part because of his fear of the devil and the Ku Klux Klan, and his belief that he had graduated from Tuskegee and Harvard.[23] Though this patient undoubtedly suffered from neurosyphilis—the Wassermann and other diagnostic tests confirmed the condition—the mention of his fear of the Klan as a delusion at best suggests white physicians' lack of awareness of a cultural context in which a Black man might legitimately fear the Klan in Indianapolis in the late 1920s. Even as Drs. Bruetsch and Bahr considered treatment of Black patients important to science, and physicians carefully noted race in the medical records, the biases of medical staff pervaded patient interactions.

Dr. Bruetsch, like other malaria therapy researchers, made observations that both built on and contributed to a long history of interpreting data on the basis of scientific racism.[24] Despite changes in psychiatric thinking after World War I, psychiatrists persisted in their fundamental belief in racialized differences between Black and white madness.[25] With regard to the experience of neurosyphilis and malaria therapy, this belief in racially different types of madness generally took two forms. First, the wrongheaded assumption that Black patients did not experience neurosyphilis meant that some patients who suffered from neurosyphilis were likely never diagnosed or treated.[26] Lack of access to medical care, too, meant that Black men and women afflicted by general paresis were likely significantly undercounted and untreated. Second, researchers including Dr. Bruetsch rather quickly concluded that malaria therapy did not work for Black patients; this "medical" observation appears to have led to both under- and overtreatment.

Regarding undertreatment, in their research notes and annual reports, Drs. Bruetsch and Bahr regularly suggested that malaria therapy did not work effectively for Black patients. As Bahr noted in 1930 in his assessment of their collective research work over the previous five years, "Some cases are immune to inoculated malaria and this is especially true of the colored patients."[27] The doctors made this conclusion despite the fact that patient records demonstrate that at least some Black patients did indeed respond to tertian malaria (a commonly used strain of malaria caused by *Plasmodium vivax*) with high fevers even in the early years of the experiment, and that at least some white patients failed to respond to tertian malaria.[28] But their assumptions about race as biologically coded influenced the way they made their observations. Although Drs. Bruetsch and Bahr were not alone in making this claim, they appear to have been among the first neurosyphilis researchers to do so. In the process, they revived older medical speculation about potential racial immunity to malaria.[29] Historian Margaret Humphreys has written about the malariologist Mark Boyd, who conducted research at a Florida state mental institution and began recording similar observations in his diary in 1931, publishing an article with a colleague two years later that highlighted their "discovery" of racial immunity.[30] But by that time, CSH was already eight years into its malaria therapy research, and Bruetsch and Bahr had begun speaking and writing about their observations years earlier.[31] Meanwhile, Tuskegee hospital director Dr. Eugene H. Dibble Jr. and a research team were also writing about the alleged "immunity" of Black patients to the tertian strain of malaria in the early 1930s.[32] Thus, Drs. Bruetsch and Bahr were among the first of a growing group of syphilis researchers who contributed to a national conversation about supposed racial "immunity" to malaria that relied on biological assumptions about race.

With Bruetsch and Bahr as white doctors in positions of authority, their medical observations carried significant weight, even as their whiteness protected them from segregation and racial hostility. By contrast, Tuskegee's Dr. Dibble—Black physician and medical director of John A. Andrew Memorial Hospital—operated within a more conscribed and tenuous authority. Dr. Dibble supervised the study that withheld treatment from Black men suffering from syphilis, even as he also oversaw and encouraged research on neurosyphilis at the local Veterans Hospital, which ultimately did treat patients with a combination of malaria and penicillin in the mid-1940s.[33] Thus, even as the US Public Health Service experiment at Tuskegee's Andrew Memorial Hospital prohibited the treatment of the Black men enrolled, the Tuskegee Veterans Hospital treated seventy Black men with the experimental combination treatment. Susan M. Reverby argues that Dr. Dibble's seemingly contradictory support for both the infamous study and the malaria therapy experimentation should be understood within the context of his overarching desire to bring health care to long-neglected Black communities that struggled to survive in the violent and segregated South.[34] By contrast, at CSH there is no evidence that either Dr. Bruetsch or Dr. Bahr held any particular commitments to racial progress. On the contrary, the doctors at CSH prioritized scientific progress, and the science that shaped their understanding of psychiatry as well as the scientific knowledge that they produced together relied on the belief in a fundamental difference between Black and white illness.

Drs. Bruetsch and Bahr believed that their Black patients were immune to malaria, and as such they believed malaria therapy to be ineffective (or less effective) in treating these patients. Perhaps surprisingly, this belief led not just to instances of undertreatment, but also instances of overtreatment with malaria therapy. Despite their belief in racial immunity, Dr. Bruetsch often repeatedly inoculated patients with the same malaria strain when they did not show the good response he was looking for (high fevers). This meant that Black patients (whom Bruetsch presumed to be immune) were often double treated with malaria therapy, and sometimes even given additional forms of treatment, despite the dangers this may have posed. Several patients (primarily, but not exclusively, Black women and men) were treated with malaria therapy two or more times over the course of several years. This, despite the fact that the treatment, which carried its own set of risks as outlined in chapter 3, did not seem to help.[35] It is perplexing that Dr. Bruetsch double treated patients he believed to be immune. Perhaps the second inoculation (and even for some, the third and fourth), like the first in many cases, was guided by Bruetsch's ongoing interest in more research data. In addition to the double inoculations, some patients were treated with malaria plus additional risky treatments. For instance, a middle-aged man was treated with both malaria and diathermy (the use of electrical currents to produce heat in the body) and died days later. In the autopsy Bruetsch noted the unusual appearance of the heart muscle and wondered whether the changes he observed "might not have been caused by the diathermy treatment."[36] Presented with challenging cases, including those who did not respond as expected to malaria therapy, Dr. Bruetsch continued to experiment, whether by trying the treatment again or by adding in new treatments.

Meanwhile, in Tuskegee, after researchers observed what they believed to be racial immunity to tertian malaria, they switched to "quartan malaria," which they argued was more successful. As Dr. Dibble reported in 1932, "through the exhaustive study and research of our Assistant Clinical Director, it was found that by the use of the quartan strain of malaria—a foreign strain to which the Negro patient had not developed an immunity—gratifying results could be obtained . . . and beneficial results began to be achieved."[37] Though the report clearly made biologically determined assumptions about race, it nonetheless found a solution to the problem that doctors perceived. In Florida, too, Mark Boyd found success by switching to the *Plasmodium falciparum* strain of malaria. This switch, which would seem to have clearly demonstrated that Black patients did not in fact have blanket immunity to malaria, unfortunately encouraged the use of *P. falciparum*, which was far more dangerous and deadly than tertian malaria, meaning that Black patients were subjected to even riskier treatment.[38]

In 1940, prompted by their communication with doctors at the Tuskegee Veterans Hospital, physicians at CSH received their first "citrated quartan malaria blood" and immediately inoculated "four colored and 4 white patients."[39] This evidence of direct collaboration with neurosyphilis researchers in Tuskegee suggests the degree to which CSH was embedded in the national medical conversation about race, syphilis, and experimental treatment. It also perhaps suggests the degree to which research priorities motivated patient treatment, again blurring the lines between the two. This is most evident in the fact that in 1944 both Dr. Bruetsch and Dr. Dibble (on behalf of the Tuskegee Veterans Hospital) participated in the National Research Council's trial of penicillin and the malaria-penicillin combination treatment. In fact, Dr. Bruetsch, who was proud of his (and CSH's) inclusion in this national research experiment, took special care to ensure that the men and women who were enrolled in the study were only treated with either penicillin alone or the penicillin-malaria combination. One older man's file, which noted his treatment with penicillin provided by the National Research Council, contained a handwritten note from Bruetsch, saying, "do not treat this patient with any other anti-syphilitic therapy.... Patient belongs to study carried on under the auspices of the national research council."[40] The use of the word *belongs* underscores the ways that mentally and physically disabled women and men at CSH supplied the raw material for the production of knowledge.

The deeply embedded scientific racism of the day shaped the way that Drs. Bruetsch and Bahr understood and articulated their medical observations, even as their conclusions contributed to that scientific racism.[41] Scholars Karen E. Fields and Barbara J. Fields describe the long-standing historical practice of confusing "folk thought" with genetic research as one example of the process of belief formation they term *racecraft*. As a concept, racecraft helpfully highlights the ways that ordinary, unquestioned activities contribute to racial formation and racism. Psychiatry, institutionalization, and experimental treatment reinforced racism through the "mundane routine" of practicing medicine.[42] The preexisting belief in racial medical differences may have guided the day-to-day practices of CSH's malaria therapy research project, but the daily practices themselves—the "mundane routine" of malaria treatment—contributed to the construction of these beliefs. The decades-long malaria therapy research project at CSH shaped the way those who were involved with it thought about race, disability, and "normalcy."[43]

The observations made by malaria therapy researchers like Dr. Bruetsch produced medical knowledge that continued to play a role in predominant medical theories throughout the twentieth century. In fact, it seems likely that their observations laid the groundwork for medical theories about sickle cell anemia developed in the 1950s.[44] And yet the conflation of genetics with race both resulted from and contributed to racecraft. The fact that Drs. Bruetsch and Bahr (among others) pinned medical conclusions on perceived racial difference reveals the historical processes of racecraft at work in both the context of a midwestern city and the broader national medical discourse. The practice of malaria therapy functioned as one of these ordinary-seeming processes that ultimately contributed to racialized thinking. Perhaps it was precisely in the day-to-day research activities of injecting malaria into critically ill patients and then observing, writing, and drawing conclusions on the basis of perceived race; perhaps it was all of those activities "nested in mundane routine" that stitched together the fabric of medical knowledge and race such that racecraft became invisible, just as Fields and Fields claim that it was designed to be.[45] With the malaria therapy research occurring as it did at the same time as, and in communication with, the Tuskegee experiment, the "mundane routine" of medical research at a state mental institution both reflected and reinforced biological assumptions about race in medicine that contributed to the same racial stereotypes and medical racism as the more infamous southern study did. In the process, patients' disabled minds and bodies provided the research to make it so.

Gender Ideology and "Successful" Malaria Therapy

Gender ideology, too, was both reflected in and constructed through the process of institutionalization and the malaria therapy research project. Perhaps the most obvious way that institutionalization at CSH was gendered is demonstrated by the physical separation of women and men in the CSH housing facilities: the men's building and the separate women's building, also known as Seven Steeples. This sex segregation was common at state mental institutions across the nation during the interwar era.[46] Beyond this physical separation, gendered assumptions regarding women (and men) are evident in the patient files, which reflect and extend gendered biases of the time. In addition, Bruetsch and Bahr's definition of "successful" malaria therapy treatment relied on gendered assumptions regarding usefulness, ability, and productive labor.

At CSH women and men occupied separate physical spaces, a gendered categorization process that began immediately upon admission. Intake forms, which were often completed by a family member or other

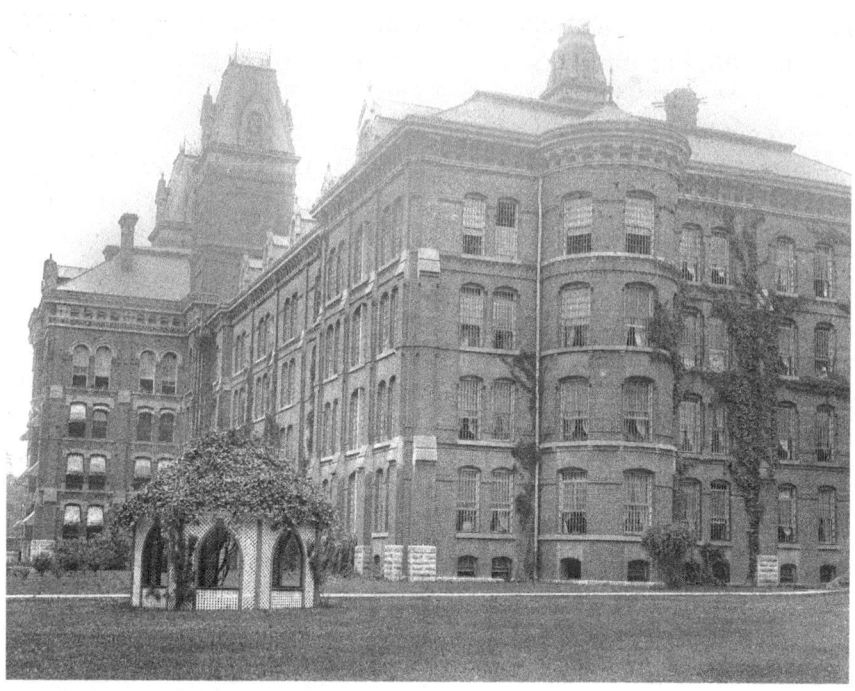

Seven Steeples, the women's building. Central State Hospital Collection, 2005447. Courtesy of the Indiana State Archives.

individual responsible for committing the patient, included lengthy sets of questions regarding the patient's health, family, work, and sexual history, and gendered differences in the ways these questions were answered are evident. For instance, whereas men's employment was typically specifically labeled, women's employment was predominately noted as "housewife"; this was true even when a closer look at the individual history would suggest that the woman had worked outside the home at some point and in some capacity. The regular use of "housewife" as a stand-in for women's labor seems to at least partly reflect the fact that most women dying from general paresis were middle-aged mothers, whose domestic responsibilities in their homes were foregrounded in their files.[47]

Additionally, though intake forms asked multiple questions about women's sexual histories, the responses to these questions were often quite limited, especially as compared to those found on men's intake forms. Women (or the individuals committing them) frequently answered no in response to whether they had venereal disease, whereas male patients seemed much more inclined to answer yes. This, despite the fact that laboratory tests regularly confirmed syphilis. One woman strongly denied having syphilis, even though her "blood is four plus wasserman," conclusively positive.[48] Perhaps women feared answering questions about sex and sexual history. Perhaps such questions forced them to relive their shame. After all, the general public linked their illnesses to sexual promiscuity and immorality. Venereal disease marked women as degenerate.[49] Of course, it is equally possible that this woman and others like her genuinely did not know that they had syphilis. Not only do women's files contain fewer acknowledgments of known syphilis infection, they tend to have fewer remarks about sexual experiences than do men's files. Intake notes casually describe men's pre- and extramarital sexual histories with comments such as, "Masturbated some. Played around a little before he was married"; "He masturbated as every boy does but not to excess. . . . Before his marriage his morals were rather loose"; and "Evidently he has engaged in venereal excess."[50] By contrast, women's sexual histories were often rather thin, sometimes just stating, "nothing known about sexual life before marriage."[51] Taken together, the intake notes reflect predominant gender assumptions of the time, but they also may indicate the particular ways that women experienced institutionalization and treatment for neurosyphilis. Women who suffered from neurosyphilis may have lacked knowledge about their illnesses; they likely felt shame or embarrassment; they may have felt scared.

As discussed in chapter 3, isolation, loneliness, embarrassment, shame, and loss shaped many patients' experiences of institutionalization, and this seems particularly true for women. Intake notes included intrusive assessments of women's bodies that revealed gender biases. As one historian has noted, psychiatric interest in the "every day" combined with the biological realities of syphilis created a context in which physicians felt entitled, even obligated, to pepper patients with intrusive questions about sex and the domestic realm.[52] At CSH physician patient notes include assessments of women's bodies as well as their behavior. For instance, one physician recorded his female patient's breasts as "large and flabby."[53] Yet another indicated that a twenty-four-year-old female patient "does not have proper domestic relations with her husband since her attack of influenza two years ago." And a third referred to a woman as a "wench," noting in the physical exam that the patient's "gait and features are typical for that of a wench of about forty years of age."[54] Such descriptions reveal gendered expectations regarding femininity, as well as stereotypes about women's sexuality and promiscuity associated with madness. Admission to CSH was likely not only challenging but also potentially embarrassing for women suffering from the physical devastation and the emotional stigma caused by neurosyphilis. Women patients were also more likely than men to be labeled "hysterical" and "high strung" in their behavior.[55] Given that a small minority of women continued to be institutionalized for "hysteria" at this time, this description problematically confused the neurosyphilis diagnosis, seemingly arbitrarily injecting physicians' gendered moral judgments.[56] Women were also more frequently compared to children than were men. One female patient was described as looking "filthy in appearance, rather wild expression in her eyes . . . she wanders about the country at night, playing along the public highway like a child," and yet another woman "must be cared for like a baby."[57] Just as they did racialized biases, intake notes and patient files reflected gendered biases on the part of physicians and medical staff that hint at women's experiences of shame.

At CSH, Drs. Bruetsch and Bahr defined success as the ability to return patients to work. Annual reports frequently referred to patients as "workers," suggesting that this was the ultimate "good" outcome. Further, gender and gendered expectations about labor shaped assumptions regarding what successfully cured looked like. In its attempts to cure all patients—not just those suffering from paresis—CSH administration sought to make "industrial" occupation a key tool in the rehabilitation of the mentally disabled. As Superintendent Bahr regularly noted in annual reports, the institution recognized "the great importance of furnishing our patients suitable employment," and as such, "we undertake, as far as possible to give them some useful work to accomplish." According to Bahr, those patients who were physically and mentally able were regularly engaged in work within the institution, "in the wards, shops, laundry, mattress shop, tin shop, dining rooms, kitchens, lawns, farm and garden, and in various other activities of the hospital."[58] Employment within the institution marked an important form of rehabilitation, and employment outside the institution reflected its ultimate success. In 1931 Bahr argued for the success of malaria therapy as a cure by highlighting several paretic patients who had been treated as part of the very first group and who were now "back at their former occupation, doing satisfactory work and earning the same wages as before the outbreak of general paralysis."[59] At CSH, neurosyphilis cure meant discharge from the hospital *and*, importantly, a return to work.

This excitement over the prospect of malaria therapy returning patients to work (including reproductive work for women) suggests one way that the treatment may have offered an alternative to typical eugenic solutions to degeneracy. Drs. Bruetsch and Bahr framed the malaria therapy as a valuable "service to the community," noting that successful discharge and return to work saved the state of Indiana a significant financial sum in final care costs.[60] This concern for community financial savings mirrored the claims made by eugenics reformers as discussed in chapter 1. Drs. Bruetsch and Bahr further noted that a shorter duration of paretic symptoms frequently led to better outcomes among patients. According to the doctors, those patients who had only exhibited symptoms of general paresis for between one and six months were far more likely to find success with the malaria therapy, with 50 percent of this group becoming "able to resume their former occupation." Among the more severe cases—those patients who had been experiencing general paresis for two years or longer—only 3 percent successfully returned to work. Of this more severe group, women accounted for the bulk of those cured, with cure being determined by their ability to return to taking "care of their household duties."[61] Researchers thus framed malaria therapy as successful at least in part due to its ability to return a small portion of men and women to gendered expectations of family and work life.

The goal of returning patients to work in an out-of-hospital setting relied on a gendered division of labor that prioritized women's work in the domestic realm. Indeed, malaria therapy "success" stories depended on the restoration of physical "ability" to perform gendered productive labor. This notion of "success" within the institutional context, relying as it did on generalized assumptions about the connection between "ability" and mental and physical health, also demarcated those considered "disabled" as "abnormal," existing outside the proper boundaries of gendered productive labor. The language of malaria therapy success regulated "normalcy" from an ableist and gendered perspective.[62] Unfortunately, the reliance on an ability to return to work as the major criterion for successful cure obscures any knowledge of the content or the texture of the lives of these supposedly "cured" patients.[63] Once patients were discharged their conditions were not followed or updated unless they returned to CSH. As it turns out, however, some of these "cured" patients did in fact relapse and return to the hospital, where they became once again disabled and "unfit."

Ironically, even as researchers saw women's return to household work outside the institution as a marker of success, within the institution some medical staff exhibited less tolerance of patients' penchant for work and usefulness, especially if those patients seemed to reach beyond their socioeconomic status. One twenty-four-year-old woman seemed to take pride in her daily work at the hospital. As recorded by medical staff, "Because she was allowed to do little chores about the ward she had the idea that she would receive a nurses uniform and would be paid on Saturday for her work." The staff notes reveal some irritation about this patient, observing that she "assumes unauthorized responsibility, judging herself to be a nurse."[64] The physical boundaries of the institution effectively established a different set of standards regarding productive work and ability. Although successful malaria therapy could transport a person back to the landscape of "normal," within the confines of the institution one's status as "patient" always relegated women and men to the realm of "abnormal," regardless of their productive capacities.

Reproduction and Eugenics

By the end of her life, the only thing that Mabel Smith remembered was that she had given birth to a baby who had lived for five minutes. She had no memory of her parents, her siblings, or her two husbands. But she knew that she had given birth.[65] Mabel held the loss of her child close, still present in the depths of her impaired mind, even in the last days of her life. The indelible mark of this memory on the mind of a woman who was experiencing severe mental impairment powerfully suggests the impact (whether positive or negative) of pregnancy and childbirth on women's lives. And yet upon admission to CSH both women and men lost the ability to make any choices about their reproductive lives. From the moment of admission these mentally "defective" patients were perceived as unfit for reproduction. In 1907 Indiana became the first state in the nation to pass a eugenics law that allowed for the sexual sterilization of institutionalized women and men.[66] Whereas "successful" malaria therapy may have offered an alternative to eugenic sterilization—after all, it held the potential of returning madwomen and madmen to their "proper" productive and reproductive roles—the failure of malaria therapy set the stage for further institutional intervention into their reproductive futures.

Women's reproduction was deeply affected by medical incarceration at CSH, thus providing yet another example of the ways that neurosyphilis and malaria therapy produced gendered consequences. Some women arrived at CSH pregnant; other women became pregnant or infected with syphilis while at CSH; some women were furloughed to give birth; and still other women were ordered sterilized during their institutionalization. In all cases, medical authorities made decisions about women's reproduction without their input. These institutional decisions both responded to and further shaped prevailing assumptions about "normalcy," "ability," and "fitness," all of which reflected and sustained hegemonic gender ideologies and practices.

Dr. Bruetsch and other neurosyphilis researchers accidentally "discovered" that malaria therapy was safe for pregnancy when they inoculated several pregnant women without first realizing that they were pregnant. At CSH Dr. Bruetsch inoculated a pregnant fifteen-year-old girl, who developed ten malarial fevers "without any complications." Just three months later, the teen "gave birth to a healthy baby." Other researchers, too, inoculated women only to later discover that they were pregnant. And as Bruetsch recalled, one researcher by the name of "Rosner" intentionally treated "eleven pregnant women with the very purpose to ascertain how inoculated malaria is tolerated by these patients and gather facts on the effect of malaria upon the fetus."[67] Based on this experimentation in conjunction with the accidental cases, Dr. Bruetsch concluded that "pregnancy does not constitute an unusual risk, in particular since most of the pregnant patients belong to the younger age group in which fatal complications due to malaria are less frequently encountered."[68] Ironically, however, this assessment did not account for the riskiness of malaria therapy in general. Additionally, no follow-up studies were conducted on babies; successful delivery was determined solely by a live birth. Nor were any studies conducted regarding the long-term health and wellness of pregnant women suffering from neurosyphilis who were malaria-treated and required to give birth.

Nonetheless, Dr. Bruetsch believed that the successful inoculation of pregnant patients shifted the calculus about whether pregnant women suffering from general paresis should have their pregnancies terminated. Bruetsch noted that medical wisdom at the time stressed the "disastrous effect of gestation upon the course of paresis," advocating for the "interruption of the pregnancy" in order for doctors to more successfully treat the woman experiencing paresis.[69] But Bruetsch argued that his (and others') safe inoculation of pregnant women countermanded that medical impetus to abort pregnancies. Experimenting on pregnant women, Dr. Bruetsch and other researchers produced medical knowledge about their reproduction that ultimately left them out of the reproductive decision-making process.

Perhaps somewhat ironically, even as CSH made it possible for pregnant women who suffered from neurosyphilis to give birth, the hospital frequently sent them home to do the gendered reproductive work of childbirth. In fact, being furloughed to give birth seems to have been one of the indicators of "successful" malaria therapy treatment, with several women's files noting furloughs for childbirth. At least one autopsied patient was noted to have been pregnant during her malaria therapy treatment, which took place at another local institution, Robert W. Long Hospital. The woman was furloughed for the birth and delivered a live child at the end of that pregnancy. Several years later, the woman gave birth again during yet another furlough, this one from CSH. This time, she returned to CSH after her furlough "in worse condition, practically helpless," and she ultimately died.[70] Although CSH permitted (perhaps even encouraged) women to leave the institution for childbirth, it seems that these women often experienced physical or mental decline in the aftermath, returning to CSH. And, at least in this case, the work of childbirth during the woman's furlough appears to have wrecked what remained of her physical health.

Although in 1921 Indiana briefly reversed course on its infamous 1907 eugenics law (which had allowed the sterilization of the mentally ill and criminals), finding it unconstitutional, the state passed a new eugenics law in 1927, in the wake of the US Supreme Court decision *Buck v. Bell*. This new law, which focused almost entirely on curbing the reproductive capacities of those individuals deemed mentally unfit by the state, stayed on the books until 1974. The state of Indiana sterilized approximately 2,500 men and women without their consent across those five decades.[71] Indiana was not alone in its embrace of eugenics; thirty US states as well as dozens of countries passed similar eugenics legislation. From sexual sterilization to marriage restriction laws, Indiana devoted multiple decades of the twentieth century to attempting to direct and shape the reproductive lives of disabled women and men.[72] Although Indiana primarily targeted the "feebleminded" for sterilization, with the overwhelming majority of these sterilizations occurring at the Fort Wayne State School and the Muscatatuck State School, some sterilizations nonetheless occurred at state mental hospitals.[73] At CSH, annual reports for the years 1935–38 included information on sterilization surgeries performed. Over the course of that brief period, twenty-seven female and eight male patients were sterilized, with more than three times as many women receiving surgery than men (and two of those women dying because of their surgeries).[74] Although it is unknown how many of these patients suffered from general paresis, at least a handful of the files of those who died from the disease include notes regarding sexual sterilization. One patient file includes a court record from 1937 recommending this procedure: "the court finds the best interest of society and of said [patient] will be served by his sexual sterilization."[75] The decision to sterilize the mentally disabled because it was in "the best interest of society" highlights the ways Indiana's embrace of eugenics overlapped with the state's efforts toward "progressive" social reform and the "progress" of modern medicine.[76]

In addition to implementing sexual sterilization, Indiana became one of several states to institute a requirement for syphilis testing to acquire a marriage license. As discussed in the introduction, CSH superintendent Bahr strongly supported this effort, seeing it as crucial to help ease the state's burden of syphilis care. The purpose of these "eugenic marriage laws" was to prevent syphilitic men and women, who were deemed medically unfit, from reproducing.[77] Although these efforts were framed within the context of the urgency of the public health drive to curb congenital syphilis, legal practices to control reproduction nonetheless meant that women and men who suffered physical and mental impairments caused by neurosyphilis were positioned outside the boundaries of "normal" civic society. It is also perhaps worth noting that restrictive marriage laws sought to protect future babies rather than women from the dangers of venereal disease, even though many women appear to have contracted syphilis from their husbands. What did this mean for women's experiences of sex and marriage in the interwar era? Ironically, even as most of the attention given to fighting venereal disease during the Great War targeted women as vectors of infection who threatened soldiers, at state institutions like CSH, husbands appeared to pose the more significant risk to their (often unknowing) wives.[78] Mabel

Smith likely acquired syphilis from her first husband. Her records note that no one in her family had been diagnosed with syphilis, and she had no additional family history that might suggest congenital syphilis. This, combined with her young husband's early death from cerebral hemorrhage as well as her infant child's death, suggests syphilis contracted through sexual intercourse with her then boyfriend.[79] For Mabel, as with so many other women, the impact of acquiring syphilis changed everything about her life, even as it also tragically shortened it.

Conclusion

Unfolding as it did within the context of the 1920s medical and social reform embrace of eugenics, the malaria therapy experiment played a multifaceted and sometimes contradictory role. On the one hand, medical conclusions made by neurosyphilis researchers based on race both reflected and contributed to scientific racism. And yet on the other hand, "successful" malaria therapy seemed to counter the ideas of hereditarianism embedded in eugenics by offering the potential return of patients disabled by neurosyphilis to lives of productive and reproductive labor. Although Indiana passed the first eugenics law in the nation, the state would be outpaced by California in number of sterilizations performed after this law was deemed unconstitutional in 1921. Not coincidentally, it was during this time period that CSH began its malaria therapy experiment, nearly a full decade before many state mental institutions began using this and other more radical medical procedures.[80] Malaria therapy may have initially offered the hope of rehabilitating women and men suffering from incurable general paresis. But as it became clear that most malaria-treated patients did not recover from their illnesses, malaria therapy looked less like a magic bullet and more like one of the many radical therapies that generated medical knowledge. In the process, malaria therapy took on a constitutive function, not only reflecting but also constructing racial and gender ideologies of the time that intersected with dominant assumptions about disability and normalcy.

CHAPTER 5

Dying from Neurosyphilis and the Silencing of Disability

On February 27, 1931, at 10:25 p.m., Mabel Smith let out her last breath. She was twenty-eight years old. In life she had stood five feet six and a half inches tall, but in death her body was "emaciated." She died in the medical ward at Central State Hospital (CSH), where just weeks earlier she had been inoculated with malaria, and so her death return recorded the cause of death as "general paralysis of the insane." For two weeks prior to her death, Mabel had also suffered from a "trophic sacral ulcer," and though her death certificate noted this as a "significant contributing condition," it did not cause her "terminal condition."[1] The skin lesion on Mabel's lower back just above her tailbone was likely caused by her bedridden state in the last weeks of her life. The bedsore, possibly infected or abscessed, was a direct result of tissue damage caused by her inability to move. Malaria therapy had clearly failed in Mabel's case. And though nothing in Mabel's patient file mentions malaria as a contributing cause, it nonetheless seems possible, even likely, that malaria inoculation hastened her death. In October and November 1930 physicians recorded Mabel's walk as "staggering," but by February 1931, in the aftermath of malaria therapy, Mabel no longer got out of bed. At 9 a.m. the day after Mabel's death, Dr. Prenatti inspected Mabel's body, noted that the family had refused autopsy, and signed the death return.

Shame, embarrassment, and secrecy accompanied both venereal disease and institutionalization. Neurosyphilis combined these two stigmatized experiences, such that the people who suffered from it were left not only physically and mentally devastated, but also shrouded in secrecy, in a desperate effort to avoid stigma and shame. The shame spread from the individual experiencing disability to their family members, who sometimes made health-care choices that were predicated on their desire to escape the painful emotion.[2] As Dr. Max Bahr noted, some families even removed their dying relatives from asylums right before their deaths so as to elude the shame of a syphilis diagnosis as the official medical cause of death.[3] Other families endured their shame privately, silencing the experiences of neurosyphilis and institutionalization. The deadly combination of venereal disease and insanity became entirely unmentionable. It is perhaps not surprising, then, that death from neurosyphilis, like death from the malaria therapy treatment for it, was also unmentionable.

Mabel Smith was silenced in life and in death. The family shame accompanying her transgressive sexual behavior and her acquired mental and physical disabilities gave way to additional shame in the wake of her institutionalized death. This chapter argues that institutionalized death and its aftermath, which were shrouded in shame and secrecy, contributed to constructions of normality that rendered women and men suffering from sexually acquired mental impairments unworthy of memory. Death and its aftermath accelerated the process of "de-lineating" disabled family members that had begun with institutionalization.[4] In addition to de-lineating families, the regular medical practices of autopsy and dissection further stripped disabled women and men from public memory, erasing their embodied lives.

Autopsy played an important role in the malaria therapy research project at CSH, and also more broadly in the continuing twentieth-century evolution of medical knowledge and science. As such, Superintendent Bahr and Dr. Walter L. Bruetsch continued to produce medical knowledge from the bodies of their deceased disabled patients. Autopsy and dissection, which were viewed by CSH administrators as "customary" practices, produced medical knowledge about neurosyphilis that ultimately relied on institutional access to disabled and marginalized patients. As such, these after-death practices contributed to the malaria therapy research project's constructions of gender, race, and disability. Disabled patients who had served as research data in life continued to do so in death.

Death and the History of Dissection and Autopsy

American perceptions of death shifted from the nineteenth through the twentieth centuries, such that by the 1920s Americans increasingly avoided discussing death. The romantic ideal of "the beautiful death," which had dominated the early nineteenth century, suggested that there was a "good" and "respectable" way to die, which included being at home in one's bed surrounded by family. But increasing medicalization over the course of the nineteenth century contributed to changing perceptions of death, as the process of dying moved from the home to the hospital, where it became a medical event to be overseen by medical experts. Death became both invisible to the public and gradually absent from public conversations. Historian Philippe Ariès has claimed that by the early twentieth century, Americans began to deny death's existence, considering death itself to be "dirty," something that should not be witnessed or discussed.[5] Meanwhile, as modern medicine succeeded in saving individual lives, death seemed like a failure on the part of the individual who died. Death in general, and death by syphilis-induced insanity in particular, became perceived as a shameful, unnatural failure.[6]

At CSH, disabled women and men who died were often quietly buried on-site. The shame of mental disability gave way to the shame of death, which went largely unmemorialized. Over the course of its long history, multiple different pieces of land at CSH appear to have been used as the institution's cemetery, with little documentation regarding who former patients were and where they had been buried. A 1995 "cleanup" of the cemetery and existing grave markings, which failed to follow original documentation, further muddled the history.[7] The lack of care in memorializing death in the 1920s and 1930s reflects the lack of respect given to disabled patients during their institutionalization and treatment in life.

As much as Superintendent Bahr liked to think of CSH as a hospital that cured insanity, in most years, well over 100 patients died, representing as much as 10 percent of the hospital's total population at any given time. Between 1924 and 1940, 2,468 women and men died at CSH.[8] Given that as many as 24 percent of newly admitted patients at CSH suffered from syphilis, it is fair to surmise that many of these deaths may have resulted from complications of neurosyphilis.[9] In his effort to elevate the research department at CSH, Superintendent Bahr appears to have made a special effort to secure permission for autopsy from patients with known and available family members; this included patients suffering from neurosyphilis. By the 1920s Indiana state law permitted educational autopsy only with family consent.[10] Many files of those patients who died at CSH include either records of autopsy or copies of letters from Superintendent Bahr requesting permission for autopsy. Although officials may not have felt the need to request patient or family consent to *treat* patients, they clearly worked hard to secure the necessary consent and permission to *autopsy* patients who died.

Autopsy represented scientific research in its purest sense; after all, once an autopsy was needed, there was no longer any hope for treatment or cure. Thus, unlike other aspects of the malaria therapy project, which served as both treatment and research, autopsy was entirely about research. The purpose of a postmortem examination of the body was to confirm a cause of death and further advance medical knowledge and science. Except for the fact that autopsy required access to a dead body, a body to which a human individual had been attached just seconds before death transpired, autopsy could conceivably be considered entirely unrelated to the individual experiences of institutionalized disabled patients. But, given its important role in the larger malaria research project at CSH, autopsy is entirely relevant to these experiences. At least in part because of the ambiguity embedded in the uncertain moment between life and death, because of the very attachment of a live, breathing human individual to what became a lifeless corpse, because of the way that surviving Americans thought and felt about the dissection of dead bodies at the time, and because of the power dynamics involved in whose bodies were dissected, the story of autopsy in the malaria therapy research project represents its vital closing chapter.[11]

Throughout the eighteenth and nineteenth centuries, Americans strongly opposed the postmortem dissection of bodies, perceiving it as an intolerable assault on the body and fearing the spiritual consequences of disturbing the physical remains of the dead.[12] Historians have identified the Civil War as a turning point in nineteenth-century ways of understanding and dealing with death in the United States. This turning point hinged on the unpleasant reality of dead and maimed bodies "littering" battlefields. The proliferation of corpses and body parts in need of tending contributed to the practices of cremation, embalming, and dissection becoming more acceptable.[13] That said, a power imbalance existed with regard to which bodies were considered permissible for legal dissection. This power imbalance in the treatment of the dead mirrored inequalities embedded in the social fabric of life, such that even as Americans gradually became more accepting of the idea of autopsy and dissection, marginalized bodies continued to be the target of most of those practices.

As the Civil War prompted new thinking about how dead bodies would be tended, mid-nineteenth-century America simultaneously saw the establishment and proliferation of medical schools, which increasingly relied on cadavers for anatomical instruction, setting up a growing conflict over the use of dead bodies for medical science.[14] Prior to the passage of anatomy laws, only the bodies of deceased criminals could be legally dissected, and yet their numbers could not keep pace with the growing demand for cadavers, as the needs for anatomical instruction increased alongside the explosion in medical schools. As several historians have noted, the unbalanced tension in supply and demand led to the illegal practice of "body snatching," the plundering of graves, particularly those of the poor and indigent, for profit.[15] This practice of grave robbing was also racialized, with African American graveyards besieged by "resurrectionists" and other body snatchers.[16] By the late nineteenth century, grave robbers regularly and intentionally targeted African Americans in their efforts to provide medical schools with the cadavers they sought. Medical schools, though often complicit in this illegal and unethical practice, frequently preferred to plead ignorance about the origins of their corpses for study.[17]

As the public concern about body snatching grew, an increasing number of states passed anatomy laws, which sought to expand legal permission for dissection to include any "unclaimed" body.[18] Although anatomy laws sought to end grave robbing, these laws increased the supply of "legal" bodies for dissection by simply relabeling the use of marginalized bodies as "legal." In practice this meant that anyone who could not afford to pay for burial risked losing their deceased loved one's body to medical science. It also meant that disabled bodies—those already marginalized and often abandoned at state institutions—were considered less worthy of protection from medical school dissection than were bodies considered normative. Several historians have noted that even if state anatomy laws brought nineteenth-century grave robbing to an end, the inequities embedded in these laws resulted in the continued exploitative use of predominately Black, poor, and marginalized bodies for dissection.[19] Indeed, the passage of anatomy laws legalized the dissection of institutionalized women and men who were unclaimed by family members. Their institutionalized lives were already perceived by many as disposable; in the wake of anatomy laws, women and men deemed insane had even fewer protections from unwanted autopsy, further demarcating their disabled lives as "abnormal," existing outside the boundaries of the perceived civic community.

The state of Indiana passed its own anatomy law in 1879 in response to a high-profile case of body snatching. Shortly after his death and burial, the body of US congressman John Scott Harrison, the son of President William Henry Harrison, was found at the Ohio Medical College, eliciting public outrage and a call for reform.[20] And yet, although Indiana's anti–grave robbery legislation may have been prompted by the growing concerns of the white upper class, which feared the potential traumatizing theft of their loved ones' bodies, in reality, it was people of color, the poor, and the marginalized who had reason to be fearful of the loss of bodily autonomy in death.[21] In 1879 the *Indianapolis News* interviewed an anonymous medical student who described the ways bodies were plundered from graves in Indiana to provide for the educational needs of medical schools. The student claimed that resurrectionists regularly visited the "old cemetery and the country graveyards" to procure bodies, which were sold to the medical schools for twenty-five dollars each. The student further noted that "at least two-thirds were colored subjects; they are more easily procured than white ones, and when we are discovered there isn't such an infernal row raised."[22] In a detached manner, the white student revealed both the persistence of racism in death, and the ways that power and inequality intertwined with racism to make death's aftermath more dangerous for those who had been marginalized in life.

Although state anatomy laws offered protection to those (primarily white) individuals who could afford private burial, they simultaneously ensured that medical science continued to rely on the deceased bodies of the marginalized and dispossessed.[23] The 1879 Indiana law stated that any dead body in a state, county, or city institution that remained "unclaimed" after twenty-four hours was permitted to be used for dissection and scientific examination. Just over two decades later, a 1903 law created the State Anatomical Board to oversee the distribution of unclaimed bodies to medical schools.[24] And yet, despite these legal changes, which ostensibly brought about the end of illegal body snatching, legal dissection still relied on access to marginalized bodies. During the first half of the twentieth century, as one historian concluded, "dissection remained a humiliation imposed on social outcasts."[25]

In addition to the fact that anatomy laws permitted *legal* dissection of marginalized bodies, *illegal* dissections also continued to occur. In November 1931 Indianapolis coroner Fred W. Vehling was accused by several families of conducting "curiosity" autopsies on deceased loved ones whose bodies had ended up at the City Hospital morgue. Relatives argued that autopsies had been conducted illegally on the bodies of people who had died from natural causes. In the absence of criminal suspicion, the law prohibited autopsy of bodies for educational or "curiosity" purposes without an approved permit from the city board of health that demonstrated family consent.[26] In several cases families noted that no permit had been obtained. In other cases, relatives claimed that they had been coerced into giving permission for autopsy, noting that Vehling had threatened to withhold death certificates if an autopsy was not agreed to.[27] Between these alleged cases of illegal dissection and the legal dissections of "unclaimed bodies" that were permitted by the anatomy laws, it is clear that Indiana residents who lacked power and resources faced a potential loss of bodily autonomy in the wake of their deaths. Institutionalized disabled patients were particularly vulnerable in this way.

Autopsy as Part of the Malaria Therapy Research Project at CSH

At CSH autopsy was practiced as a routine part of the malaria therapy research project. Even as the general American public may have been slow to appreciate the importance of the dead human body to the production of medical knowledge, medical researchers were acutely aware of the need for corpses in the race to advance science. Indeed, as scholars have noted, medical schools desperately needed the dead.[28] Certainly this awareness undergirded much of the research at CSH, where Superintendent Bahr noted in the 1940 annual report that the aim of the pathology department "has been to study the autopsy material of insane patients in the same scientific spirit as autopsy material is evaluated in a general hospital."[29] Prioritizing pathology and research, Bahr sought to make these departments at CSH the centerpiece of its success, referring to this research as the "heart of the medical work."[30] Annual reports regularly cataloged the numbers and types of research specimens collected through autopsy at CSH. In the process, segments of disabled bodies were separated from the individual people that they had been in life; the dead bodies of women and men suffering from neurosyphilis morphed into disembodied specimens for study. These specimens, removed from the larger context of life and its accompanying story, were carefully labeled, preserved, numbered, and studied.[31] This process of dissecting disabled bodies in order to create medical knowledge further demarcated "normative" civic life from that which was considered abnormal, dangerous, and threatening. Perhaps more than any other feature of the malaria therapy experiment at CSH, the story of autopsy leaves the clear impression of patients as research data.

In addition to making a national and international name for themselves in research, Drs. Bruetsch and Bahr also sought to make CSH indispensable to medical education in the state of Indiana. As such, the research conducted at CSH took place in close collaboration with the Indiana University School of Medicine, with Bruetsch and Bahr—both of whom also held faculty positions—regularly offering clinics and lectures at CSH for Indiana medical students.[32] Bahr summarized the importance of this work, noting among the many benefits CSH offered to the medical school that it provided "a large and fully equipped pathological laboratory with amphitheater for lectures and clinics, furnishes appropriate and abundant material for research and investigation, and also affords an excellent opportunity for teaching the Science of Mental and Nervous Diseases."[33] Autopsies formed an essential component of this educational relationship, with medical students observing Dr. Bruetsch (who served as both pathologist and director of research) perform autopsies on deceased patients in CSH's large laboratory amphitheater.[34] Indeed, Superintendent Bahr frequently championed this aspect of Bruetsch's work in the annual reports, noting CSH's "Class A status," meaning that the "hospital is recognized by the American Medical Association as one of the hospitals having the necessary qualifications for the training of residents in psychiatry."[35] A 1927 Indiana legislative act required that all medical practitioners demonstrate at least two years of training at an institution "where instruction includes dissection of the human body."[36] With its Class A status, CSH's pathology department played a crucial role in fulfilling the requirements of medical training in Indiana. As such, autopsy at CSH was vital to both its research and its teaching programs. And given that the malaria therapy experiment remained the primary focus of CSH research over the course of several decades, a significant number of the autopsies conducted between 1924 and 1945 dealt with neurosyphilis and malaria therapy.

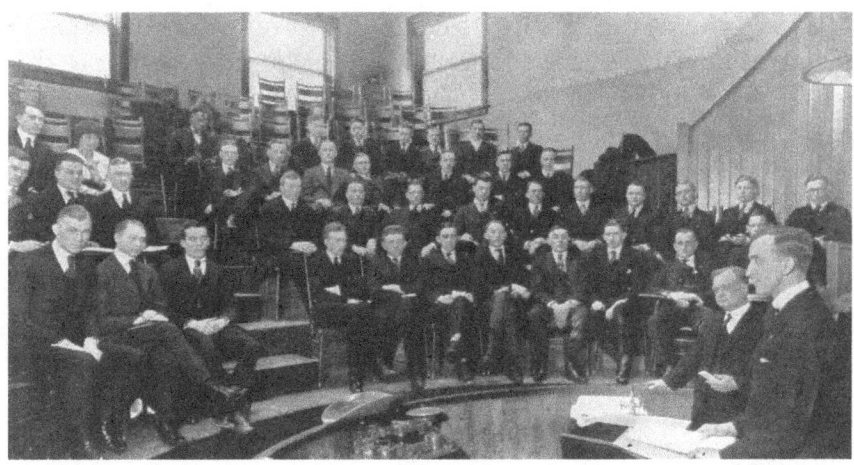

Medical students in the amphitheater of the old pathology building. Courtesy of the Indiana Medical History Museum.

Just as treatment and research overlapped at CSH in patient care, so too did autopsy and dissection overlap in the aftermath of death. Although CSH regularly used the word *autopsy* to describe the postmortem examination of bodies, the distinction between autopsy and dissection seems muddled at best. Scholars note that autopsy has historically been considered distinct from dissection in that the purpose of autopsy is to determine a cause of death, whereas the purpose of dissection is to advance medical learning. Claiming that the latter resulted from structural violence and marginalization while the former did not necessarily carry the same social stigma, one anthropologist writes that "autopsies marked an individual as important enough ... to warrant an investigation of their death."[37] Although this distinction between autopsied bodies and marginalized dissected bodies is helpful—particularly for the consideration of medical intentions—such a clear demarcation does not adequately capture the historical reality of the malaria therapy research project's reliance on autopsy and its consequences for disabled women and men.

From 1925 to 1945 the institutional context in which people suffered neurosyphilis at CSH meant that marginalized patients experienced medical experimentation followed by routine autopsies that fundamentally resulted in the production of far more medical knowledge than merely the cause of an individual's death. CSH records regularly referred to autopsy, rather than dissection, which would seem to suggest that the primary objective was to determine a cause of death. But even if determining the cause of death was *one* goal of autopsy at CSH, this was evidently not the *only*, or even necessarily the *primary*, goal. Indeed, autopsies at CSH appear to have regularly included dissection, with brains (and sometimes hearts and other organs) removed, preserved, and cataloged for the express purposes of further study, both in research and in teaching. As Bahr noted in annual reports, "autopsy material" was used "extensively" in medical instruction for those who were studying psychiatry and neurology, with 5,840 "microscopical preparations... made from autopsy material" in one year alone.[38] Autopsies at CSH—including those conducted on neurosyphilis patients—produced a tremendous amount of material for medical research and educational purposes.

In addition to producing knowledge about neurosyphilis and malaria therapy, "autopsy material" generated at CSH helped make medical training for Indiana University medical students possible. Dissected human bodies and organs were carefully cataloged, labeled, and stowed in glass specimen jars, to be viewed by hundreds of medical students learning about psychiatry and neurology. Dr. Bruetsch sometimes returned to a dissected brain to conduct follow-up dissection and research months or even years after the initial autopsy.[39] In this way, disabled bodies and minds continued to produce medical knowledge long after their human deaths. Although CSH secured permissions and legal permits for these autopsies, the usage and display of disabled body parts long after death nonetheless raises questions about whose bodies were protected and how. Did family members who consented to autopsies in the 1920s and 1930s know that dissected pieces of their loved ones' brains might remain in glass jars for years to come? Did those same family members sign the consent forms under any duress or because they lacked access to private burial? Such questions, which interrogate the fuller context in which permissions for dissection were granted, could help further center the voices of the institutionalized in the story of autopsy.

Nationally, the medical display of vulnerable bodies, particularly the remains of African Americans, occurred frequently throughout the twentieth century, reflecting what scholar Harriet A. Washington calls "the final manifestation of medical racism."[40] In 2000 the daughter of Bessie Wilborn—a twenty-eight-year-old Black Georgia woman who died of Paget's disease in 1950—filed a lawsuit against the Medical

College of Georgia for having displayed her mother's disfigured skeleton in its pathology lab for half a century without her knowledge or consent. Although the Medical College insisted that it had done nothing wrong, having legally acquired the body through "donation," Wilborn's daughter had always assumed that her mother was safely buried.[41] At CSH, where the pathology lab similarly displayed organs and other human specimens for decades, it is unknown whether families of the deceased understood the potential ramifications of providing consent for autopsy or donation. The display of the disabled in death reinforced the constructions of normalcy that were made during life.

At CSH Dr. Bruetsch's lengthy pathology reports supplied far more information than merely the cause of death. His detailed reports in the files of those who died from neurosyphilis often commented on new medical observations, linking postmortem examinations to CSH's larger body of research on the disease and its treatment. Taken all together—the dissected organs, the pathology reports, and the reliance on autopsy to collect specimens to support research, education, and the production of more medical knowledge—the evidence of the use of dead bodies at CSH suggests a lack of any clear distinction between autopsy and dissection. Indeed, autopsied bodies became just as important to the malaria research project as living bodies that experienced a successful cure. Perhaps CSH preferred to use the word *autopsy* precisely because it lacked the social stigma of dissection. But with its intentional focus on becoming a national teaching and research center, even the confirmation of an individual's cause of death was ultimately made in service of education and research. The pathology department may have referred to the procedure as autopsy rather than dissection, but in the end, the result seems the same. The bodies of marginalized patients who experienced medical experimentation while institutionalized in life became the research data to support medical knowledge production in death.

Between 1924 and 1940 CSH recorded 542 autopsies completed under the direction of Dr. Bruetsch. That number represented between 13 and 50 percent of all the deaths that occurred at CSH during each fiscal year.[42] Drs. Bruetsch and Bahr clearly considered autopsy an essential component of their malaria therapy research, and as such, they consistently sought permission from patients' next of kin for autopsy. In at least one case, a patient's family members wrote to CSH requesting information about their loved one's death and about whether he had remembered anyone in the family prior to dying. The family also requested the results of the pathology report.[43] This suggests that for this family at least, autopsy ostensibly served the purpose of providing some answers regarding the cause of death. But this type of communication and query from families is lacking from most patient files. Presumably CSH may have also autopsied patients whose bodies went unclaimed, as the anatomy laws permitted, but there is no clear indication in patient records when such a situation may have occurred. Instead, patient files sometimes included copies of Superintendent Bahr's requests and reminders for family members to complete what he referred to as "the customary autopsy" form to give CSH permission to dissect the bodies of the deceased.[44]

Although few patient files contain evidence of correspondence with families, official requests for autopsy permission are an exception to this norm. In one, Bahr wrote, "On checking the records of . . . we find that the customary autopsy blank has never been signed. We ask that you sign it and return it at once so that we can complete his record." In yet another file, Bahr wrote to the county clerk in an effort to find the correct address for the patient's "correspondent." His letter began, "Dear Sir, We are very desirous of getting in touch with. . . . " This detective work was apparently successful, as the patient's family member signed an autopsy consent form that was dated just a few months after Bahr's inquiry.[45] These brief and somewhat clipped requests to families for permission to autopsy, even before the death of the patient had occurred, makes it seem as though death was not only expected, but highly anticipated. This expectation that insane patients would die during their institutionalization seemingly contradicts Bahr's more public writing, in which he often distinguished CSH as a *hospital* engaged in the *cure* of mental disease rather than a custodial institution for the hopelessly insane. The fact that autopsy permission was considered "customary" and that the permission was so aggressively pursued seems to suggest that administrators expected their mentally disabled patients to die. It further suggests that these deaths and the autopsies that followed were perceived as valuable for the malaria research goals of CSH. As such, the women and men who died of neurosyphilis at CSH quickly transitioned from individual person to research data. So rapid in fact was the transformation that one might be compelled to think that patients had really served as research data all along.

As discussed above, autopsy reports clarified diagnosis and cause of death in addition to advancing knowledge about the effects of malaria therapy and the neurosyphilis disease process. As such, these reports sometimes produced surprising results. In fact, on several occasions Dr. Bruetsch noted that a malaria-treated patient could not be confirmed on autopsy to have had either general paralysis or the malaria treatment.[46] This is somewhat confusing, and even opens up the possibility that some patients who were believed to have been suffering from neurosyphilis (for instance because of their Wassermann test results) were misdiagnosed. In some cases, the autopsy failed to confirm the diagnosis of neurosyphilis, even though the patient had been treated with malaria therapy.[47] In one case, even the Wassermann test was reported as negative, and yet still the patient had been treated with malaria.[48] As with the arbitrary nature of treatment discussed in chapter 2, through autopsy, the imprecision of diagnosis and treatment sometimes became obvious. For instance, an immigrant woman who did not speak English was treated with malaria therapy, and yet her pathology report noted that the autopsy did not look like that of a typical paretic; rather, Bruetsch noted that "in the aorta, there is not the least sign indicating syphilis."[49] Is it possible that the language barrier resulted in medical staff failing fully to understand the woman's condition and potentially even mistreating her with malaria? Or perhaps the language barrier made it even easier for medical staff to take advantage of a vulnerable inmate, treating her with malaria regardless of her condition. This case and others like it provide additional evidence regarding the uneven application of malaria therapy treatment criteria, and the consequences of that uneven application.

Each individual body that was autopsied became a collection of its parts, consisting of yet more data points to be observed and studied. Bruetsch's postmortem studies of the bodies of his patients project a sense of curiosity and wonder about the bodily impacts of neurosyphilis and malaria therapy. Whereas patient files provided significant detail on the pre-syphilis lives of women and men, pathology reports noticeably omitted any description of the person, instead focusing on the body and its many separate parts. As is common with a pathological report, each organ was described in detail. Ultimately, however, the existence of pathology reports within the patient files serves as a reminder of the fact that the women and men who died at CSH contributed to the larger syphilis research undertaking. In several autopsy reports Dr. Bruetsch noted the time of death as less than one hour prior to the time of autopsy. In one case the time of death was noted as 6:35 p.m., and the autopsy began at 7:00 p.m. As a reader, I find it hard not to feel the weightiness of this decision to cut into bodies so soon after death. In such cases Bruetsch began his autopsy report with the words, "the body is still warm."[50] One might think that the general public would have had reservations about the rapidity of these dissections in the aftermath of death. After all, the fear of being buried alive was a concern that permeated the psyche of many Americans as early as the founding of the nation.[51] Such fears led some in the late nineteenth century to lobby for a waiting period of at least one to three days before dissection took place.[52] That said, from a medical research viewpoint, autopsy was best conducted as soon after death as was possible. Presumably modern science and medicine assumed that the expertise of the pathologist was enough to ensure that a patient was indeed dead. More than anything, however, Dr. Bruetsch's uncanny ability to slip so easily from provider of malaria therapy to detached pathologist and researcher suggests his overarching commitment to his medical research.

Constructing Disability through Death and the Silences That Follow

During fiscal year 1931, when Mabel Smith died, CSH conducted only twenty-four autopsies, representing just 19 percent of the deaths that year. In the annual report Superintendent Bahr explained that this low rate of autopsy was due to the six-month-long absence of Dr. Bruetsch, "who utilized this time for study at the Universities of Berlin, Vienna, and Paris."[53] Autopsy was clearly a primary component of Bruetsch's work as pathologist—at times he appears to have been the only pathologist on staff qualified to complete dissection—but it was also a regular and expected part of the CSH experience during the interwar period.[54] That said, Mabel Smith's body was not autopsied. Instead, her parents came to collect her dead body, and they buried her privately. Though she was not buried at nearby Crown Hill—a cemetery reportedly reserved for white and upper-class Indianapolis residents—Mabel's private burial in a Catholic cemetery serving the area nonetheless protected her dead body from the dissection table.[55] Mabel's family "refused" autopsy, though the death return does not make it clear which family member (her husband, Arthur, or one of her parents, Michael or Katherine, perhaps?) made the decision. Perhaps CSH would not have had the resources to provide an autopsy even if its staff had wanted one, as Mabel died during the six-month period when Bruetsch was in Europe. Perhaps Mabel's loved ones declined CSH's customary autopsy request because of their Catholicism.[56] Or perhaps they had the troubled feeling held by many Americans that dissection represented an assault on the body. Perhaps, like many Americans, they did not appreciate the medical usefulness of autopsy.[57] Or perhaps they simply wanted to bury Mabel (and had the means to do so at the Catholic cemetery) and put the story of her venereal disease and insanity behind them. It is difficult to say just how many families declined autopsy. It is equally difficult to identify how many patients did not have next of kin to ask. Rather, what seems clear is that the dead whose bodies ended up on Dr. Bruetsch's autopsy table originated from a group of people generally deemed unworthy in the larger society. Over the course of several decades, the hearts and brains and other organs of people who had died of neurosyphilis were removed from their bodies and preserved in jars for research and education, and more research.[58] In fact, these disabled bodies, which had been marginalized in life and dissected in death, became foundational to the production of medical knowledge,

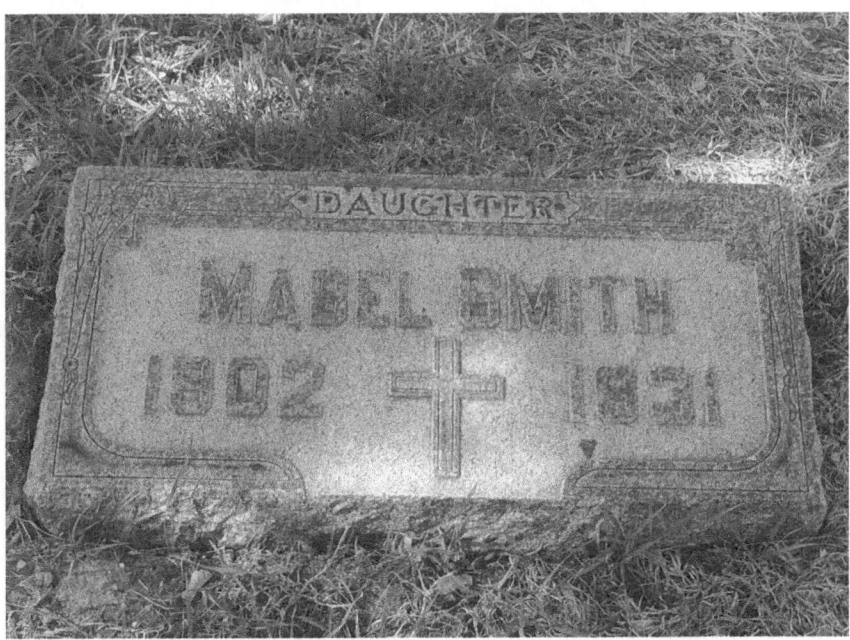

Mabel Smith's headstone. Photograph by Christin L. Hancock, 2017.

to the education of medical students, and to the professional prestige and success of both Dr. Bruetsch and CSH.

In his explanation of the early nineteenth-century era of the "beautiful death," Philippe Ariès notes that the final moments of togetherness, the last "communion" between the dying and those people that the dying person was about to leave behind, marked a death as good and "beautiful." By contrast, when death became "dirty" and "medicalized," the beauty of this last communion was destroyed, removing "the great privilege of the dying."[59] According to Ariès, the medical profession—which had taken over death and made it invisible—could have stepped in for the missing community, but instead isolated death "in the scientific laboratory and the hospital, from which the emotions would be banished," ultimately responding with silence and leading the community "to be ashamed of death."[60] If such a scenario played out amid death in the general population in the twentieth century, the silencing and shame that resulted was a mere fraction of that which greeted the deaths of institutionalized patients who suffered and died from neurosyphilis. Patients at CSH often died alone, with no community and no hope for any final communion with loved ones. They died in the women's building or the men's building or the infirmary. After death, some of their bodies found their way to the scientific laboratory, where they were dissected for science and medical knowledge. Their presumed sexual promiscuity, their madness, their institutionalization, and their deaths all invited shame. And families responded to that shame with a silence that persisted for generations.

Conclusion
Revisiting Mabel, Dismantling Shame

Unlike what happened with most patients at Central State Hospital (CSH), Mabel Smith's parents came to collect her body in the aftermath of her tragic death. Burying her past alongside all the hopes and dreams they might have held for their oldest child, the Daltons covered Mabel's grave with a headstone that read simply "Daughter." In their grief and shame, they erased her transgressive behavior, her sexuality, her brief motherhood, and her two marriages, and reclaimed Mabel for themselves, greeting future queries about their eldest daughter with a silence that persisted for generations. Meanwhile in the archives of CSH, Mabel Smith became malaria therapy patient #253, her place in the nearly forgotten line of Dr. Walter L. Bruetsch's research work.

The shame that accompanied venereal disease and its resulting madness imprinted itself on the physical bodies of Mabel and hundreds of other women and men in the form of visible illness, acquired disability, and institutionalization. In utilizing a feminist disability studies approach that centers the embodied experiences of those suffering from neurosyphilis, this book argues for the critical central role of *people* in the stories of medical history. More than merely a history of disease and experimental treatment, this is a story of relationships. It is a story of relationships between young lovers and their family members; relationships between those considered disabled and those considered able-bodied; relationships between institutionalized patients and their care providers; relationships between physical bodies and interior selves; and, perhaps most fundamentally, relationships between individuals who experienced shame and their communities, whose efforts at enforcing certain expectations and behaviors ultimately resulted in shaming. As such, I hope the book offers a framework by which centering disability history helps us think more critically and more holistically about medical history and its gendered, human, and relational ramifications. Additionally, in re-lineating my own disabled family member—not only weaving her back into my family history, but also situating her within a larger public history of disability, shame, and madness—I hope the book serves as a template for recovering previously erased and silenced stories and voices to help provide a fuller accounting of family and community history alike.

Mabel's story and the stories of hundreds of others who were treated with malaria at CSH also reveal the ways that the overarching institutional commitment to medical progress overlooked the very real human experiences of pain and fear and isolation. Researchers' single-minded focus on "cure" obscured patients' experiences of treatment, disregarding their physical and emotional pain. As a potential remedy for the devastation caused by neurosyphilis, malaria therapy also offered the promise of a "cure" for the shame and degeneracy that accompanied the diagnosis. But success—relying as it did on the premise of returning women and men to their expected productive roles in society—meant that this "magic bullet" both reflected and contributed to gendered and racialized ideologies of the time. It also meant that when malaria therapy failed, as it did for so many, those who died continued to be marked as "abnormal," "unfit," and "shameful." Malaria-treated women and men who nonetheless died had failed to redeem themselves, bringing additional shame to themselves and their surviving family members.

Malaria therapy played a multifaceted, sometimes contradictory role in the history of eugenic thinking. On the one hand, malaria therapy replicated and contributed to eugenic thinking and medical racism. And yet on the other hand, "successful" malaria therapy offered the promise of rehabilitation, an outcome generally not perceived as possible by the eugenic belief in hereditarianism. Ironically, when the treatment proved effective, the success called into question the very eugenic thinking that had spurred it into being. Occurring as it did at the same time as the infamous Tuskegee study, malaria therapy as practiced at state institutions across the nation is a critical but largely overlooked piece of the story of medical research and experimentation on marginalized women and men. The inverse side of the history of experimental *nontreatment*, malaria therapy reveals a fuller account of this history by highlighting the ways that medical racism was also embedded in the everyday practices and routines of experimental *treatment*. As such, the telling of this history reminds us that institutions—including those dedicated to medical care and scientific progress—have historically reflected inequalities of power and contributed to communities' social expectations regarding that which is considered "normal." These inequities have long-lasting and deeply impactful human consequences. This history, then, also importantly reminds us to question the ways our current institutions of medical care, particularly those entrusted with the care of the most marginalized members of society, reproduce inequalities of power and shape social expectations in the process.

Dr. Walter L. Bruetsch and Malaria Therapy

In spring 1958 Dr. Walter L. Bruetsch wrote to the newly appointed dean of Johns Hopkins Medical School, Dr. Thomas B. Turner. "Possibly you remember me from the days when we both were interested in syphilis, malaria treatment, etc.," Bruetsch began his missive.[1] Dean Turner had remembered Bruetsch "very well indeed," recalling "with a great deal of pleasure, the days when we had strong common interests in syphilis, malaria treatment and related problems."[2] Although by the early 1950s penicillin had proved itself superior to both malaria and the malaria-penicillin combination that Bruetsch and others associated with the National Research Council had studied in the 1940s, the researchers who had invested decades of their professional lives studying malaria therapy and neurosyphilis continued to think fondly of their years devoted to this scientific research. Throughout his older age, Bruetsch continued to practice his love of medical research, moving on to new studies. Sending yet another reprint of new research to Dr. Turner in 1968, this time on "the collagen diseases," Bruetsch included a handwritten note: "After the conquest of syphilis I found a fascinating new field here."[3] These fond remembrances of the heyday of malaria therapy research suggest not only a pride in their presumed success in vanquishing syphilis, but also a nostalgia for those heady research days. In these small details there is a sense that perhaps despite Bruetsch's description of his new work as "fascinating," he was never quite able to replicate the exciting times of malaria therapy.

Mabel Smith may have vanished after her death in 1931, but Dr. Bruetsch, the researcher, continued to oversee the malaria therapy treatment of neurosyphilis at CSH for nearly two more decades. In the process, Dr. Bruetsch made a name for both himself and the Indiana hospital, staking a leadership claim in international medical research, and creating knowledge from the lives and deaths of women and men disabled by neurosyphilis. At CSH Dr. Bruetsch and Superintendent Max Bahr hoped to bring an end to a devastating medical scourge that carried enormous social and economic implications. In the quest for medical progress that dominated the era, women and men spiked high fevers again and again, until, in some cases, malaria seemed to successfully kill the syphilis spirochete.[4] And in other cases, it killed the patient.

And yet, while researchers like Bruetsch may have justified their work by highlighting its therapeutic nature, the history of the experimental treatment itself tells a fuller story, one that hints at all the social flaws wrapped up in the human interaction between medical provider, researcher, and patient. Embedded in the quest for "progress" were biased assumptions about disability and normalcy that fit neatly within the increasingly popular eugenic thinking of the day, which dominated much of medical thought as well. Also embedded in this quest were all the local social values and their attending inequities of gender, race, and poverty that pervaded an interwar midwestern city. At CSH, Dr. Bruetsch seemed to relish the inclusion of all patients in malaria treatment, which provided more material for his research. Although racism and sexism did not exclude patients from malaria treatment, they nonetheless shaped the way doctors viewed their patients, the ways they defined "success," and the medical knowledge that was generated.

Dr. Bruetsch functioned as a medical researcher in a historical and cultural moment when medical research was prized, and individual clinicians' expertise was particularly valued. He and other medical leaders may have believed that the "beneficence" that malaria therapy provided to patients marked by fatal illness absolved them of any ethical concerns. And yet this slippage between treatment and research provided the context in which more than one thousand marginalized women and men who suffered from neurosyphilis became the research data on which both the institution and the researchers constructed their professional standing. Researchers at CSH in Indianapolis portrayed malaria therapy as a cutting-edge experimental project, and yet also as just one of several forms of modern treatments offered by a leading psychiatric institution. Patients who suffered from the debilitating physical and mental effects of neurosyphilis were largely overlooked; they were critical to the research and yet left out of the story.

Mabel Dalton Ward Smith

When Michael and Katherine Dalton buried Mabel's body at the Holy Cross and Saint Joseph Cemetery—the Catholic cemetery serving the south side of Indianapolis, which included their parish of St. John the Evangelist—they embraced Mabel as their daughter, even as they also began a generations-long process of silencing her full life story. The Daltons responded to their own grief and shame about Mabel's illness and death, which had transgressed the boundaries of "normal," by locking this shame away in silence. Historian Peter N. Stearns has noted that although the meaning and experience of shame is shaped by historical context, the pain of shame is "always real."[5] It is challenging to tease out the pain caused by grief and that caused by shame. In many ways they overlap; psychologist Silvan Tomkins noted that death of a loved one can in fact cause shame, a type of pain that can be felt "as a defeat, as intolerable loneliness, as a temporary distancing between the self and the other, as a poignant, bitter-sweet longing."[6] Perhaps the Daltons' silence stemmed from a combination of the intense parental grief of losing a child (which in itself can cause shame) and the shame caused by Mabel's sexual transgressions, which appear to have led to a cascading series of shameful events. Even though Mabel's unwed pregnancy occurred during a time of generally diminishing shame culture nationwide, the stigma associated with women's sexual immorality persisted in Indiana in the 1920s, and in fact, such shame largely persisted throughout the twentieth century.[7] It is perhaps not surprising, then, that parents experiencing such grief and loss may have continued to face a culture of shame throughout their own lives.

Six years before Mabel's death, the Daltons had arranged for the burial of her first husband, Irvin, in the Catholic cemetery. Perhaps Irvin's family could not afford the burial, or perhaps the Daltons' concern and compassion for their young, widowed daughter motivated their involvement. And yet, though they apparently arranged and paid for the burial, they did not mark Irvin's final resting place with a headstone. Perhaps the cost was too much, or perhaps they felt that they had done enough given the circumstances. When Mabel died in 1931, Michael and Katherine buried her in the same plot as Irvin, covering the two with a headstone that honored Mabel alone.[8] Calling her "Daughter" only, the Daltons quite literally covered up Mabel's illegitimate pregnancy and her first marriage. Mabel's younger brother Tom was fourteen years old when she died alone at CSH. In December 1940 Tom Dalton married Rosemary Dolan at St. John the Evangelist. Over the course of the next several decades, they raised ten children—five boys and five girls—in a skinny, two-story white house on South Meridian Street, less than five miles from CSH and just one mile north of Holy Cross and Saint Joseph Cemetery. The children grew up on the south side of Indianapolis surrounded by their living aunts and uncles and their fellow parishioners. Although their childhood home stood not far from the insane asylum where their Aunt Mabel had been injected with malaria and died, and nearby the grave where she was buried, she and her story remained absent from their lives.

The Dalton family erasure paralleled a larger historical erasure of Mabel's story as well as the stories of women and men like her who suffered and died from neurosyphilis. The erasure affected not only individual families, but also larger cultural expectations regarding gender, sexuality, and meanings of ability, disability, and "health." The historical silencing of these stories perpetuated both family and cultural biases against disability and madness.[9] Additionally, the erasure of women's stories of neurosyphilis and malaria therapy treatment has (even if unintentionally) lent itself to buttressing the mistaken notion that women's historical experiences of madness have always *only* been a result of the very real psychiatric tendency of pathologizing women who transgressed gender boundaries. Revisiting Mabel and others like her is my attempt to stitch them back into the historical record. It is my attempt to provide a counterbalance to the power imbalances that shaped so much of their life and death experiences. In centering their embodied experiences, I hope their stories help dismantle the shame that has historically attached itself so thoroughly to disability, madness, and women's sexuality.

Notes

Introduction

1. Mabel Smith patient file, CSH patient records, Indiana State Archives (ISA).

2. The term *paretic*, which was commonly used by health professionals at the time, referred to one who was suffering from "general paralysis of the insane" (GPI). In the 1920s and 1930s, *general paralysis of the insane, general paresis*, and *paresis* were regularly used diagnostic terms to describe neurosyphilis. As Gayle Davis explains in her history of GPI in Scotland, "by the 1920s, GPI formed the core of a new wider disease category, neurosyphilis, an umbrella term which grouped together those diseases held to be late manifestations of syphilis that had infiltrated the nervous system, including tabes dorsalis, syphilitic insanity and cerebral syphilis." See Davis, *The Cruel Madness of Love*, 16. In this book, I use the terms *neurosyphilis, general paralysis, general paresis*, and *paresis* interchangeably.

3. Mabel Smith patient file, CSH patient records. Because Mabel Smith is my great-aunt, I have chosen to use her real name. All other evidence cited from patient files of the CSH archives is made anonymously, out of respect for the privacy of the women and men who were institutionalized there.

4. CSH superintendent Dr. Max Bahr noted in 1917 that neurosyphilis was responsible for the first admissions of at least 20 percent of patients at CSH. See Bahr, "Nervous and Mental Diseases in Relation to Public Health," 7–8.

5. Brandt, *No Magic Bullet*; Davis, *The Cruel Madness of Love*; Parascandola, *Sex, Sin, and Science*; Quétel, *History of Syphilis*.

6. Stearns, *Shame*, 76.

7. Catherine Kudlick historicizes the concept of "cure" in "Social History of Medicine and Disability History," 112.

8. "Success" rates varied over time and by hospital, but in the first five years of treatment in the United States, researchers generally identified 25–30

percent success rates. The now common practice of using randomized controlled trials (largely considered the gold standard in medical research) did not begin until the late 1940s.

9. Davis, *The Cruel Madness of Love*, 16.

10. For a historical description of the anguish caused by malaria inoculation, see De Kruif, *Men against Death*, 261.

11. Garland-Thomson, "Feminist Disability Studies," 1557. For more on feminist disability studies and madness, see Donaldson, "Revisiting the Corpus of the Madwoman," 93.

12. My general use of the term *woman* is meant to be expansive and inclusive, referring to anyone who defines themself as a woman. My description of patients at CSH as women and men is based on medical records and other archival sources that categorized each patient as "male" or "female," and then segregated them as such.

13. Dyck, *Facing Eugenics*; Lombardo, *A Century of Eugenics in America*; Lombardo, *Three Generations, No Imbeciles*; Lombardo and Dorr, "Eugenics, Medical Education, and the Public Health Service"; A. M. Stern, *Eugenic Nation*.

14. See Stearns, *Shame*, ix–xi. Theorist Eve Kosofsky Sedgwick notes that shame makes a "double movement . . . toward painful individuation, toward uncontrollable relationality." See Sedgwick, *Touching Feeling*, 37. Thanks to Molly Hiro for pointing me toward Sedgwick and Silvan Tomkins. See Hiro, "How It Feels to Be without a Face."

15. Historian John Demos writes, "To be sure, the audience is sometimes imagined, not real; but the sense of being watched, of being exposed and unfavorably scrutinized, is central either way." See Demos, "Shame and Guilt in Early New England," 70.

16. Demos, 70.

17. Stearns, *Shame*, 3–4.

18. Fink, *All Our Families*, ix–xix, 18.

19. My thinking on historicizing shame is indebted to the work of Heather Brook Adams and Peter N. Stearns. See Adams, *Enduring Shame*, 1–28; Stearns, *Shame*, 1–9. My use of the phrase "all our families" is a reference to Jennifer Natalya Fink's beautifully written book with the same title. See Fink, *All Our Families*.

20. Jennifer Natalya Fink restores to her own family lineage her disabled cousin and a second relative who were born with Down syndrome and cut out of the family. In my own extended family, while neither Down syndrome nor aging was treated as shameful (to the contrary, family members experiencing disabilities associated with these conditions were embraced), sex outside of marriage as well as mental and emotional pain that interfered with "normal" life were considered shameful, even sinful. See Fink, *All Our Families*, 51.

21. Rembis, *Defining Deviance*.

22. Fink, *All Our Families*, xix.

23. Theorist Silvan Tomkins described shame as what is experienced when "one wishes to look at or commune with another person but suddenly cannot because he is *strange*, or one expected him to be familiar, but he suddenly appears *unfamiliar*." Quoted in Sedgwick, *Touching Feeling*, 35 (emphasis added). See also Frank and Wilson, *A Silvan Tomkins Handbook*, 5.

24. Braslow, *Mental Ills and Bodily Cures*, 71; Braslow, "The Influence of a Biological Therapy on Physicians' Narratives and Interrogations."

25. Humphreys, "Whose Body, Which Disease?"; Humphreys, *Malaria*; Gambino, "Fevered Decisions"; Reverby, *Examining Tuskegee*.

26. See, e.g., Pemberton, "The Curious Case of the 'Professional Hemophiliac,'" 239.

27. Michael Rembis writes that "one of the central tenets of... mad studies" is "to highlight the voices and experiences of the psychiatrized or otherwise 'mad identified.'" See Rembis, "The New Asylums," 142. Mad studies scholars like Geoffrey Reaume have advocated for more centering of the voices of those who experienced madness and disability. See, e.g., Reaume, *Remembrance of Patients Past*; Reaume, "Mad People's History." An early attempt to highlight institutionalization from the perspective of the women who experienced it was undertaken by scholars Jeffrey L. Geller and Maxine Harris in 1994. They gathered and edited twenty-six firsthand accounts of asylum experiences dating from 1840 to 1945. See Geller and Harris, *Women of the Asylum*, 1–10.

28. Kim E. Nielsen calls on "ethical historians" to treat institutional sources "carefully, tenderly, compassionately, and fully aware of how they came to be created." See Nielsen, "The Perils and Promises of Disability Biography," 25–26. For more on the problematic nature of "authoritative" sources, see Richards and Burch, "Documents, Ethics, and the Disability Historian," 162–63.

29. Richards and Burch, "Documents, Ethics, and the Disability Historian," 162, 166.

30. Disability scholar Kim E. Nielsen advocates for disability historians to visit the site of our biographical subjects in order to experience our own "embodied" response to space and material culture. See Nielsen, "The Perils and Promises of Disability Biography," 32.

31. Nielsen refers to this visitation work as "uncitable but fruitful historical research." Nielsen, 32.

32. "Symposium on Five Years' Experience with the Malaria Treatment of Neurosyphilis," *Indianapolis Medical Journal*, December 1930, CSH, Walter L. Bruetsch files, box 2, folder 7, ISA.

33. Geoffrey Reaume's work on the history of institutionalized patients' experiences provides a model for interrupting these silences. See Reaume, *Remembrance of Patients Past*, 3. Hazel Morrison demonstrates the importance of acknowledging the larger context of the creation of case notes in building a history of "patient stories 'from below.'" See Morrison, "Constructing Patient Stories," 84–85.

34. For more on "physician beneficence," see Halpern, *Lesser Harms*, 4.

35. Here I am using the term *madness* because this was the language that was used in the early twentieth century. As Erika Dyck has written, failing to use the language of the time "runs risk of forgetting the consequences of being thus labeled." See Dyck, *Facing Eugenics*, 4.

36. Donaldson, "Revisiting the Corpus of the Madwoman," 93.

37. Donaldson, 103.

38. See, e.g., Burch, *Committed*; Reaume, *Remembrances of Patients Past*; Rembis, "The New Asylums"; Erevelles, "Crippin' Jim Crow," 95; Spandler, Anderson, and Sapey, *Madness, Distress and the Politics of Disablement*.

39. Rembis, "The New Asylums," 142.

40. Susan K. Cahn refers to this sort of history as "a 'biography' of an illness and the biographies of people said to suffer from it." See Cahn, "Border Disorders," 260.

41. Anne E. Parsons, *From Asylum to Prison*; Rembis, "The New Asylums," 140.

42. As Chris Chapman, Allison C. Carey, and Liat Ben-Moshe write in the first chapter of their edited collection *Disability Incarcerated*, a scholarly study of disability and imprisonment, "Custodialism served the interests of the new helping professions. Institutions centralized treatment, research, and funding, and thus played an important role in the advancement of professionals concerned with the feebleminded." Chapman, Carey, and Ben-Moshe, "Reconsidering Confinement," 8.

43. As Erika Dyck and Larry Stewart write in their history of human experimentation, bodies became "instruments" that "made possible the credibility of scientific knowledge." See Dyck and Stewart, introduction, 6.

44. In her historical study of Native American experiences of institutionalization, Susan Burch writes, "Despite rhetoric and even intentions of settler humanitarian medical care and concern, forced psychiatric confinement . . . [has] always been—by design—carceral." See Burch, *Committed*, 16.

45. See Burch, *Committed*, for more on the carceral nature of institutionalization.

46. Brandt, *No Magic Bullet*; Braslow, *Mental Ills and Bodily Cures*, 71–90; Dowling, *Fighting Infection*; Parascandola, *Sex, Sin, and Science*; Quétel, *History of Syphilis*.

47. German physicians discovered the syphilis spirochete (bacteria) as well as diagnostic tests to confirm the disease in the early twentieth century. See Dowling, *Fighting Infection*, 91.

48. Gerald Grob writes, "at least one-third and probably one-half or more of all first admissions to state mental hospitals were cases of behavioral symptoms probably of known somatic illness." Grob, *The Inner World of American Psychiatry*, 14, and see also 3, 267.

49. Brandt, *No Magic Bullet*; Braslow, *Mental Ills and Bodily Cures*, 79; Parascandola, *Sex, Sin, and Science*, 49, 69–72. For a general discussion of the shame associated with illness, see Kleinman, *The Illness Narratives*, 158–60.

50. Lombardo and Dorr, "Eugenics, Medical Education, and the Public Health Service," 300.

51. See Jones, *Bad Blood*; Reverby, *Examining Tuskegee*; Washington, *Medical Apartheid*.

52. See, e.g., Lombardo, *A Century of Eugenics in America*.

53. Bahr, "Nervous and Mental Diseases in Relation to Public Health," 7.

54. "Citizens Sponsoring Social Hygiene Day Laud Marriage Blood Test Law," *Indianapolis Star*, January 28, 1949, Indianapolis Foundation Records (IFR), box 54, file 10, "American Social Hygiene Association, 1928–1941," University Library Special Collections and Archives, Indiana University–Purdue University Indianapolis.

55. Lombardo, *Three Generations, No Imbeciles*, 46.

56. Buckles, Guldi, and Price, "Changing the Price of Marriage," 540.

57. For more on the introduction of increasingly radical therapies during this time period, see Geller and Harris, *Women of the Asylum*; Grob, *The Mad among Us*; Scull, *Desperate Remedies*.

58. Guided by the legal parameters as defined by the 1996 Health Insurance Portability and Accountability Act (HIPAA), my research is limited to patients who died more than seventy-five years ago. Further guided by additional legal parameters set up by the Indiana State Archives Division of the Indiana Archives and Records Administration's Privacy Committee, I am committed to protecting the personal health information contained in patient records used for my research. I have done this by removing names and identifying information from my writing.

59. See, e.g., Morrison, "Constructing Patient Stories," 85; Nielsen, "The Perils and Promises of Disability Biography"; Reaume, *Remembrance of Patients Past*, 1–6; Richards and Burch, "Documents, Ethics, and the Disability Historian."

Chapter 1. Mabel Smith

1. Mabel Smith patient file, Central State Hospital (CSH) patient records, Indiana State Archives (ISA). I have chosen to refer to Mabel by her first name largely because her surname changed several times over the course of her twenty-eight years, depending on her marital status. As her last names ultimately belonged to various men (her father, and her two husbands), it seems more fitting to refer to her by her given name.

2. CSH annual report, 1949, ISA.

3. Mabel Smith patient file, CSH patient records.

4. Mabel Smith, certificate of death, Marion County (IN) Health Department, filed March 1, 1931 (in author's possession).

5. D'Emilio and Freedman, *Intimate Matters*, 194–201.

6. Geller and Harris, *Women of the Asylum*, 256.

7. See Nielsen, *Money, Marriage, and Madness*, 7.

8. Genealogical sleuthing conducted on Ancestry.com has been helpful to me in putting together dates and addresses for Mabel's life.

9. Adams, *Enduring Shame*; Rembis, *Defining Deviance*. Peter N. Stearns notes that the experience of shame has caused people to "deny" and "forget"; see Stearns, *Shame*, 4.

10. Existing records offer conflicting dates of Mabel's birth. Her death certificate from the Marion County (IN) Health Department notes her birth as July 31, 1902, while her death certificate from the CSH records her birth as July 3, 1902. Because church records show that she was baptized on July 20, I have chosen to go with the July 3 date of birth, taking the July 31 date to be an error.

11. St. John the Evangelist Catholic Church, baptism registers, book 1891–1902, #89, Mabel Katherine Dalton.

12. Payne, "Adapting the Urban Parish," 255.

13. Jacob Piatt Dunn, "Indianapolis Election of 1914 as Shown in Mayor Bell's Trial," *Indianapolis Star*, October 31, 1915, Indiana State Library (ISL).

14. "Men Indicted by County Grand Jury," *Indianapolis Star*, June 23, 1915, ISL.

15. "105 Are Freed in Election Case," *Indianapolis Star*, December 12, 1915, ISL.

16. "Bell Issues Statement," *Indianapolis News*, July 9, 1917, ISL.

17. "Men Indicted by County Grand Jury," *Indianapolis Star*, June 23, 1915, ISL.

18. "Real Estate News," *Indianapolis Star*, June 21, 1916, ISL.

19. In 1930, roughly 40 percent of American households had telephones. See Statistica, "Percentage of Housing Units with Telephones." In 1929, an Indianapolis Foundation survey reported that 53,500 homes in the city had telephones. This, in a city with an estimated total population of 411,000 people, comprising 103,689 families living in an estimated 98,600 homes, meant that Indianapolis phone ownership surpassed that of the national average. See Lies, *The Leisure of a People*, 25, 57.

20. "Charges of $3088.79 against Jacob P. Dunn," *Indianapolis News*, June 4, 1917, ISL.

21. "Police Are Investigated," *Indianapolis Star*, September 16, 1917, ISL.

22. For more on the history of eugenics, see Dyck, *Facing Eugenics*; Kline, *Building a Better Race*; Lombardo, *A Century of Eugenics in America*; A. M. Stern, *Eugenic Nation*. See also Reilly, *The Surgical Solution*.

23. US Census data for Michael F. Dalton, 1920, Indianapolis Ward 13, Marion, IN, Ancestry.com; US Census data for Michael F. Dalton, 1930, Indianapolis, Marion, IN, Ancestry.com.

24. John D'Emilio and Estelle B. Freedman found a significant increase in premarital pregnancies among the working class in the first decade of the twentieth century. See D'Emilio and Freedman, *Intimate Matters*, 199.

25. US Census data for Irvin Ward, 1920, Indianapolis Ward 12, Marion, IN, Ancestry.com.

26. In the years prior to Michael's purchase of the North Senate Street house, the Dalton family rented a house at 823 Chadwick Street. Meanwhile, in 1910 nine-year-old Irvin lived with mother Cora Ward, younger brother Raymond, and several other relatives at the home of his mother's parents, Riley and America Poole. Although Cora, who worked as a packer at a candy company, is listed in the 1910 US Census as the daughter of the head of the household (her father, Riley), Cora's two sons are recorded as "nephews." Whether Riley was grandfather or uncle to Irvin, Riley's last name was Poole, and this presumably explains where Irvin/Jack picked up his alternate name. In 1913 Cora Ward became Cora Taylor, having married a man named Ford Taylor. She and the boys then moved to Taylor's residence at 942 Chadwick, where the brothers became stepsons; their new home put them just two hundred feet from the Dalton family. US Census data for Charles E. Ward, 1910, Indianapolis Ward 12, Marion, IN, Ancestry.com; Cora Taylor, marriage registration, September 15, 1913, Indiana, US, Select Marriages Index, 1748–1993, Ancestry.com; US Census data for Cora Taylor, 1920, Indianapolis Ward 12, Marion, IN, Ancestry.com.

27. D'Emilio and Freedman, *Intimate Matters*, 195. James Glass writes that "by 1920 the Indianapolis street car system carried 126 million passengers each year." See Glass, "A Lesson in Indy's Transportation System."

28. D'Emilio and Freedman, *Intimate Matters*, 198–99; see also Peiss, *Cheap Amusements*.

29. Charting a history of Catholic opposition to eugenics, Sharon M. Leon notes that one point of overlap between Catholics and eugenicists came in the form of their mutual support of large nuclear families within a framework of "positive eugenics." See Leon, *An Image of God*, 38–39.

30. Indiana State Board of Health, Division of Vital Statistics, certificate of birth, registration #1151 8583, Ancestry.com. For more on Mabel's work history, which shifts from clerk in a furniture store to no employment, see US Census data for Mabel Smith, 1920 and 1930, Indianapolis Ward 13, Marion, IN, Ancestry.com.

31. D'Emilio and Freedman note that working-class premarital sex caused significant conflict between parents and teens/young adults. D'Emilio and Freedman, *Intimate Matters*, 198–99.

32. Stearns, *Shame*, 1, 76–77. For more on the history of churches using shaming as a disciplinary tactic, see Demos, "Shame and Guilt in Early New England," 71–73.

33. In her CSH patient record, Mabel recalled having given birth to a baby who lived only five minutes. Mabel Smith patient file, CSH patient records. The birth (and death) is confirmed by Indiana State Board of Health, Division of Vital Statistics, certificate of birth, registration #1151 8583, Ancestry.com.

34. Irvin's death certificate records his death as being caused by cerebral hemorrhage. Because this was a known symptom/outcome of neurosyphilis, and because doctors often avoided using the word *syphilis* to mitigate shame, it would not have been uncommon for a syphilis infection to be unrecorded

on official documents. Based on the available evidence, I am speculating that he died of a neurosyphilis infection and that he passed this infection on to his young wife. Similarly, because syphilis infections frequently caused miscarriage and stillbirth, and in the absence of evidence to the contrary, I am speculating that the baby also died of congenital syphilis. On cerebral hemorrhage as indicative of neurosyphilis infection, see Merritt, Adams, and Solomon, *Neurosyphilis*, 92.

35. Entry for Mabel C. Ward, 1926 Indianapolis City Directory, US City Directories, 1822–1995, Ancestry.com.

36. US Census data for Norma Dalton, 1930, Indianapolis Ward 13, Marion, IN, Ancestry.com.

37. St. John the Evangelist Catholic Church, marriage registers, 1929, Marie Dalton and James Cormack.

38. For more on the ways that shame around premarital sexual relations affected women's reputations well into the twentieth century, see Stearns, *Shame*, 76–77.

39. Communication with Marion County Circuit Court, January 12, 2016, regarding marriage certificate for Mabel Ward and Arthur Smith, dated October 5, 1929; US Census data for Arthur and Mabel Smith, 1930, Indianapolis Ward 13, Marion, IN, Ancestry.com; St. John the Evangelist Catholic Church, baptism registers, book 1903–14, #79, Arthur Francis Smith.

40. US Census data for Arthur and Mabel Smith, 1930, Indianapolis Ward 13, Marion, IN, Ancestry.com.

41. For more on the history of European immigrants becoming "white," see Jacobson, *Whiteness of a Different Color*; Jacobson, *Roots Too*; Roediger, *Colored White*; Roediger, *Working toward Whiteness*.

42. Bailey, *From Front Porch to Back Seat*; D'Emilio and Freedman, *Intimate Matters*; MacLean, *Behind the Mask of Chivalry*, 40–41.

43. Kline, *Building a Better Race*, 10–11.

44. As Stearns notes, the South and other "regions where the Ku Klux Klan was active" were slow to abandon "honor culture," especially as it applied to sex; thus, shame persisted as a disciplinary action through the 1920s. That said, by the 1930s, sexual shaming had begun to decline even in places like Indiana. See Stearns, *Shame*, 74–77; see also Demos, "Shame and Guilt in Early New England," 70–73.

45. Lynd and Lynd, *Middletown*, 112.

46. Lynd and Lynd, 113–14. For more on fears about prostitution associated with automobiles and new commercialized leisure spaces, see Bailey, *From Front Porch to Back Seat*; D'Emilio and Freedman, *Intimate Matters*, 199–200.

47. As Michael Rembis notes, "feebleminded" women, in particular, were considered both threat and victim. See Rembis, *Defining Deviance*, 2.

48. Lynd and Lynd, *Middletown*, 113–14.

49. The 1920 US Census reported 36,524 residents of Muncie City and 314,194 in Indianapolis. See StatsIndiana, "Indiana City/Town Census Counts, 1900–2010"; Peiss, *Cheap Amusements*.

50. Lies, *The Leisure of a People*, 57.
51. Rembis, *Defining Deviance*, 5.
52. Lies, *The Leisure of a People*, 67.
53. Kline, *Building a Better Race*, 13; Rembis, *Defining Deviance*; A. M. Stern, *Eugenic Nation*, 6.
54. Lies, *The Leisure of a People*, 67.
55. Alexandra Minna Stern explains the link between "degeneration" and eugenics in the 1920s; see Stern, *Eugenic Nation*, 13–18. For more on degeneracy, see also Carlson, "The Hoosier Connection"; Lantzer, "The Indiana Way of Eugenics"; A. M. Stern, "From Legislation to Lived Experience."
56. Lies, *The Leisure of a People*, 31.
57. Lies, 57.
58. Bailey, *From Front Porch to Back Seat*, 79.
59. "Exclusive Street Invaded by Women Soliciting Nefariously," *Indianapolis News*, July 27, 1931, Indianapolis Foundation Records (IFR), box 54, file 10, "American Social Hygiene Association, 1928–1941," University Library Special Collections and Archives, Indianapolis University–Purdue University Indianapolis.
60. Parascandola, *Sex, Sin, and Science*, 49–57; S. W. Stern, *The Trials of Nina McCall*, 5. See, e.g., Brandt, *No Magic Bullet*.
61. Parascandola, *Sex, Sin, and Science*, 52–60, 69. For an in-depth history of one woman's unjust imprisonment, see S. W. Stern, *The Trials of Nina McCall*. See also Bristow, *Making Men Moral*; Jensen, *Mobilizing Minerva*.
62. Adams, *Enduring Shame*, 2–5; Stearns, *Shame*, 76–77.
63. For more on the shift underway, see Grob, *The Inner World of American Psychiatry*, 1–18.
64. A. M. Stern, *Eugenic Nation*, 18; see also Sussman, *The Myth of Race*, 43–63.
65. Appleman, "Deviancy, Dependency, and Disability," 447; Carlson, "The Hoosier Connection"; Lantzer, "The Indiana Way of Eugenics"; A. M. Stern, *Eugenic Nation*, 13–16; A. M. Stern, "From Legislation to Lived Experience." See also Reilly, *The Surgical Solution*.
66. Bahr, "Nervous and Mental Diseases in Relation to Public Health," 10.
67. *Mental Defectives in Indiana*, 9.
68. Lombardo and Dorr, "Eugenics, Medical Education, and the Public Health Service," 311. For more on the history of the committee, see Osgood, "The Menace of the Feebleminded," 264–77. See also Lantzer, "The Indiana Way of Eugenics," 32–33; Sussman, *The Myth of Race*, 43–63.
69. *Mental Defectives in Indiana*, 9, 13, 15.
70. *Mental Defectives in Indiana*, 9.
71. Dr. Walter Clarke to Mr. Eugene Foster, September 18, 1930; Dr. Walter Clarke to Dr. Frederick Jackson, September 18, 1930; Dr. Walter Clarke to Dr. C. A. Stayton, November 1, 1930; Mr. Bascom Johnson to Mr. Eugene Foster, September 21, 1932; Mr. Eugene Foster to Mr. Bascom Johnson, October 8, 1932; all letters in IFR, box 54, file 10, "American Social Hygiene Association, 1928–1941."

72. Parascandola, *Sex, Sin, and Science*, 53; S. W. Stern, *The Trials of Nina McCall*, 127.

73. Mr. Bascom Johnson to Mr. Eugene Foster, September 21, 1932, IFR, box 54, file 10, "American Social Hygiene Association, 1928–1941."

74. Dr. Walter Clarke to Dr. C. A. Stayton, Indiana Medical Society, November 1, 1939, IFR, box 54, file 10, "American Social Hygiene Association, 1928–1941."

75. IFR, box 59, file 21, "Special Appropriations, 1928, General Hospital."

76. IFR, box 59, file 11, "Admitting Department, 1928–1949"; Eugene Foster to Dr. Charles W. Myers, Superintendent City Hospital, November 30, 1937, IFR, box 59, file 13, "Anti-Syphilis"; IFR, box 59, file 20, "Psychiatric Service, 1925–1947, City Hospital."

77. Marks, *The Progress of Experiment*, 54.

78. Mabel Smith patient file, CSH patient records.

79. Kobrowski, *Fractured Intentions*, 7–8, 10.

80. Geller and Harris, *Women of the Asylum*, 256.

81. Agnew, *From under the Cloud*; for an in-depth history of Agnew, see King, *From under the Cloud at Seven Steeples*.

82. For Agnew, the presence of a woman physician made all the difference in her experience, and as a result she became a strong advocate of women's medical education, writing, "And for the sake, and in behalf of suffering woman—insane women in particular—I make an appeal to the board of trustees of every female hospital for the insane in the land, for the appointment of a woman upon their medical staff." Agnew, 151.

83. Rembis notes that the "psy discourses," and the power they wielded over the historical processes of institutionalization, played a significant role in shaping that which is thought of as both "normal" and "defective." See Rembis, *Defining Deviance*, 9.

84. Silvan Tomkins writes that shame is "felt as a sickness of the soul that leaves man naked, defeated, alienated, and lacking in dignity." Excerpted in Sedgwick and Frank, *Shame and Its Sisters*, 148.

85. As Jeffrey L. Geller and Maxine Harris note, "The mere possession of a female body was thought to increase one's vulnerability to madness, and women who could not or would not adapt to their life circumstances were especially at risk." Geller and Harris, *Women of the Asylum*, 9.

86. Rembis's conclusions about the historical constructions of disability and "deviance" are valuable in guiding an approach to a gendered history of living with and dying from a fatal disease. Rembis argues that rather than attempting to dismiss the "existence of impairment, disease, or disorder, disability scholars need to meet these accusations head-on . . . and engage in a critical analysis of the formation of the diagnostic regimes so readily deployed." Rembis, *Defining Deviance*, 147; See also Watson, Roulstone, and Thomas, *Routledge Handbook of Disability Studies*.

87. CSH superintendent Max Bahr estimated in 1917 that one in nine men and one in thirty women "who died between the ages of 40–60, died

of paresis." See Bahr, "Nervous and Mental Diseases in Relation to Public Health," 7–8.

88. Heather Brook Adams argues for the importance of understanding "shame's mutability and persistence when directed to women's unsanctioned and defiant, sexual, and fertile bodies." Adams, *Enduring Shame*, 4.

89. Geller and Harris, *Women of the Asylum*, 255–56; Lunbeck, *The Psychiatric Persuasion*, 50.

90. Appleman, "Deviancy, Dependency, and Disability," 449; Geller and Harris, *Women of the Asylum*, 258. For more on the increasing use of medical therapies during the interwar era, see Tomes, *Remaking the American Patient*, 59.

Chapter 2. Dr. Walter L. Bruetsch

1. For more on the history and development of psychiatry and the relationship between US and European psychiatric education, see Scull, *Madhouse*; Scull, *Desperate Remedies*.

2. For more on the medical model's prioritization of "cure," see Kudlick, "Social History of Medicine and Disability History," 112.

3. In his historical study of malaria therapy in California, Joel Braslow writes that "a doctor's determination that a treatment works was (and is) a social act between healer and patient so that 'nonbiological' relationships were (and are) an inseparable part of the effectiveness of a somatic treatment." I argue that this social relationship between doctor and patient is also central to understanding the experiences of those for whom the treatment did not work. Braslow, *Mental Ills and Bodily Cures*, 71.

4. Rosenberg, *No Other Gods*, 141–43.

5. Bahr, "My Fifty Years of Psychiatry," 512.

6. Bonner, *American Doctors and German Universities*, 2, 23.

7. Scull, *Madhouse*, 23.

8. Bahr, "Nervous and Mental Diseases in Relation to Public Health," 7–8.

9. As historian Gerald Grob recorded, "at least one-third and probably one-half or more of all first admissions to state mental hospitals were cases of behavioral symptoms probably of known somatic origins." Grob, *The Inner World of American Psychiatry*, 14.

10. CSH annual report, 1924, 16, 20, Indiana State Archives (ISA).

11. CSH annual report, 1924, 6, 14, 20–21.

12. Bonsett, "Dr. Walter Bruetsch, Obituary," 105.

13. Walter L. Bruetsch, naturalization records, Marion County Naturalizations, Digital Collection, ISA.

14. Bonsett, "Dr. Walter Bruetsch, Obituary," 105; "Symposium on Five Years' Experience with the Malaria Treatment of Neurosyphilis," *Indianapolis Medical Journal*, December 1930, CSH, Walter L. Bruetsch files, box 2, folder 7, ISA.

15. Bruetsch, "Max A. Bahr, M.D., 1874–1953."

16. Scull, *Madhouse*. As Andrew Scull notes, Thomas Neville Bonner was, in 1963, the first to detail this history of American medical practitioners taking postgraduate training in Germany. See Bonner, *American Doctors and German Universities*.

17. Scull details the story of American psychiatrist Dr. Henry Cotton, who, like Bahr, sought training in Germany. Cotton, who became convinced that all mental illness was caused by physical infection, performed surgical procedures that killed and severely injured thousands of patients at Trenton State Hospital in New Jersey. See Scull, *Madhouse*, 30–31; Scull, *Desperate Remedies*.

18. Appleman, "Deviancy, Dependency, and Disability," 449.

19. Dowling, *Fighting Infection*, 91.

20. Neosalvarsan soon followed; see Dowling, *Fighting Infection*, 93; Marks, *The Progress of Experiment*, 54. Over the next two decades, more arsenical compounds continued to be identified and used in syphilis treatment, including Stovarsol, a French arsenical compound that became available in 1921 and was incorporated into the CSH treatment regimen in 1931. See CSH annual report, 1932, 23, ISA.

21. Salvarsan was called 606 because it was the 606th arsenical that Ehrlich synthesized. See Davis, *The Cruel Madness of Love*, 168, 169; Quétal, *History of Syphilis*, 6.

22. Grob, *The Inner World of American Psychiatry*, 3, 14, 267.

23. Lunbeck, *The Psychiatric Persuasion*, 50; see also Tsay, "Julius Wagner-Jauregg and the Legacy of Malarial Therapy," 246.

24. Brandt, *No Magic Bullet*.

25. On the relative rarity of neurosyphilis, see Crenner, "The Tuskegee Syphilis Study," 256. According to Suzanne Poirier, "about one-third of untreated patients develop tertiary syphilis," a subset of which includes neurosyphilis. See Poirier, *Chicago's War on Syphilis, 1937–1940*, 3.

26. Brandt, *No Magic Bullet*; Dowling, *Fighting Infection*, 95; Parascandola, *Sex, Sin, and Science*; Quétel, *History of Syphilis*.

27. Cynthia J. Tsay traces the history of similar fever experiments prior to Wagner-Jauregg. See Tsay, "Julius Wagner-Jauregg and the Legacy of Malarial Therapy," 247–49. See also Bruetsch, "Julius Wagner-Jauregg, M.D."; Kampmeier, "Syphilis Therapy"; Kampmeier, "Wagner von Jauregg and the Treatment of General Paresis by Fever."

28. According to biographer Magda Whitrow, Wagner-Jauregg knew that "Hippocrates mentioned the beneficial influence of a malaria infection on epilepsy and Galen cited a case of melancholy cured as a result of an attack of quartan fever." Whitrow, *Julius Wagner-Jauregg*, 151.

29. Whitrow, 153.

30. Whitrow, 153–57; Scull, *Desperate Remedies*, 92–98.

31. Tsay, "Julius Wagner-Jauregg and the Legacy of Malarial Therapy," 249–50. As Scull notes, one of the nine died, several of those reported "cured"

relapsed, and diagnosis was uncertain in another. Scull, *Desperate Remedies*, 96.

32. Whitrow, *Julius Wagner-Jauregg*, 169, and see 159–68.

33. Tsay notes that Wagner-Jauregg's embrace of Nazism and eugenics likely accounts for his disappearance from public memory within the fields of neuroscience and psychiatry. See Tsay, "Julius Wagner-Jauregg and the Legacy of Malarial Therapy," 251.

34. Ethics and experimentation are explored in more detail in the next chapter.

35. For more on the history of whiteness in the United States, see Jacobson, *Whiteness of a Different Color*; Jacobson, *Roots Too*; Roediger, *Working toward Whiteness*; Roediger, *Colored White*.

36. Lauck, Hogan, and Whitney, introduction, xi–xiii.

37. As R. David Edmunds notes, "Most residents of Ohio, Indiana, or Illinois are unaware of the Indian people living in their midst or that these people and their forebears played a major role in the history of the region and the American nation." Edmunds, introduction, 1.

38. See Jacobson, *Whiteness of a Different Color*; Jacobson, *Roots Too*; Roediger, *Working toward Whiteness*; Roediger, *Colored White*.

39. Birzer, "Jean Baptiste Richardville," 94, 97, 104. Bradley J. Birzer notes that the Miami "had long intermarried with the Creole-French" fur traders, and thus had a long history of compromise and negotiation, but this was not acceptable to the white Anglo population.

40. As Susan Sleeper-Smith notes, for those Miami who successfully resisted the removal process, many of them did so by claiming whiteness. According to Sleeper-Smith, the tragic irony of this clever strategy of resistance, which she refers to as hiding "in plain sight," was that in 1897 the federal government terminated its tribal recognition of the Miami of Indiana on the basis of their whiteness and successful acculturation. Sleeper-Smith, "Resistance to Removal," 117, 120–21.

41. Probst, *The Germans in Indianapolis*, 90.

42. Probst, 90.

43. Probst, 147–69.

44. According to Jeffrey Helgeson, "the dominant responses to the migration empowered the forces of white working- and middle-class politics that reenergized and reshaped twentieth-century American conservatism." Helgeson, "Politics in the Promised Land," 111.

45. Helgeson, 112.

46. In 1920 the population of Indianapolis was 89 percent white. See Lies, *The Leisure of a People*, 21.

47. Sample, "A Truly Midwestern City," 130.

48. Helgeson notes that the migration itself "did not initiate racial tensions in the Midwest"; rather, "the migrants brought to the surface the aspects of the region that made it both a land of hope and a place of profound

disappointment in Black Americans' diasporic movement in search of freedom and opportunity." Helgeson, "Politics in the Promised Land," 112.

49. See Walsh, "Report of a Study of the Hospital Accommodations for Colored People in Indianapolis," 7, Indianapolis Foundation Records (IFR), box 60, file 37, University Library Special Collections and Archives, Indianapolis University–Purdue University Indianapolis.

50. In 2021 there were 619,000 deaths due to malaria globally. The overwhelming majority of these deaths were among children in African nations. See World Health Organization, "Malaria."

51. Horan, *The Story of Old St. John's*, 13–14.

52. Horan, 13–14.

53. "One Malady Casts Out Another," *New York Times*, July 7, 1925, 18.

54. CSH annual report, 1925, 23, ISA. *Anopheles* refers to mosquitos that are capable of transmitting malaria.

55. Bahr, "The So-Called Recovery of Paresis," CSH, Walter L. Bruetsch files, box 2, folder 7.

56. Saint Elizabeths Hospital in Washington, DC, was one of the earliest such institutions in the country, beginning its malaria treatment in 1922. See Humphreys, "Whose Body? Which Disease?," 55; Parascondola, *Sex, Sin, and Science*, 79; Tsay, "Julius Wagner-Jauregg and the Legacy of Malarial Therapy," 250. In a 1934 medical publication, Dr. F. J. Van Meter referred to the malaria treatment as no longer an "experiment," but rather the "standard"; see Van Meter, "Malarial Treatment of General Paresis," 366. See also Bahr and Bruetsch, "Two Years' Experience with the Malarial Treatment."

57. See Bunker and Kirby, "Treatment of General Paralysis by Inoculation with Malaria"; Eldridge et al., "Treatment of Paresis." See also Bahr and Bruetsch, "Two Years' Experience with the Malarial Treatment." For a history of malaria treatment at the Mayo Clinic, see Sartin and Perry, "From Mercury to Malaria to Penicillin."

58. Marks, *The Progress of Experiment*, 53–55.

59. Marks, 53–55. For a summary of different medical approaches in the 1920s as well as analysis of the initial malaria treatment at Saint Elizabeths, see Lewis, Hubbard, and Dyar, "The Malarial Treatment of Paretic Neurosyphilis."

60. Henry A. Bunker Jr. and George H. Kirby noted in 1925 that they intentionally avoided using arsphenamins after malarial treatment at Manhattan State Hospital "in order that we might not thereby complicate the therapeutic picture." See Bunker and Kirby, "Treatment of General Paralysis by Inoculation with Malaria," 564. Meanwhile, at Saint Elizabeths at least some patients were followed with arsphenamins. See Eldridge et al., "Treatment of Paresis," 1098.

61. Marks, *The Progress of Experiment*, 53; CSH and Dr. Bruetsch were invited to join the subcommittee of the Cooperative Clinical Group in 1937. See CSH annual report, 1937, 23–24, ISA.

62. Whitrow, *Julius Wagner-Jauregg*, 166. Margaret Humphreys claims that the vast majority of American inoculations occurred through blood injection in part because the mosquito method, which was more complicated, required the expertise of a malariologist. See Humphreys, "Whose Body? Which Disease?," 57.

63. One such anecdote was shared with the author by Dr. Martha Goetsch, Oregon Health and Science University, Portland. For an example of medical literature of the time urging caution to protect communities from malaria, see O'Leary, Goeckerman, and Parker, "Treatment of Neurosyphilis by Malaria," 307, 318.

64. Bahr, "The So-Called Recovery of Paresis."

65. Bahr and Bruetsch, "Two Years' Experience with the Malarial Treatment."

66. Bruetsch, "Why Malaria Cures General Paralysis."

67. Additionally, some of those deemed cured may have relapsed years later. For statistics, see CSH annual report, 1928, 28, ISA.

68. Paul A. O'Leary reported a 49 percent remission rate at the Mayo Clinic in 1927; see O'Leary, "Treatment of Neurosyphilis by Malaria." Henry A. Bunker Jr. and George H. Kirby reported eighteen of fifty-three patients (33 percent) showing marked improvement in 1925; see Bunker and Kirby, "Treatment of General Paralysis by Inoculation with Malaria," 566. Watson W. Eldridge and colleagues reported 32.7 percent improvement in 1925; see Eldridge et al., "Treatment of Paresis," 1099. See also Braslow, *Mental Ills and Bodily Cures*, 71–94; Tsay, "Julius Wagner-Jauregg and the Legacy of Malarial Therapy," 250.

69. Bunker and Kirby, "Treatment of General Paralysis by Inoculation with Malaria," 564; Bruetsch and Bahr, "A Study of the Mechanism of Inoculation-Malaria," 210.

70. Braslow, *Mental Ills and Bodily Cures*, 78; see also Sartin and Perry, "From Mercury to Malaria to Penicillin," 259.

71. Bruetsch and Bahr, "A Study of the Mechanism of Inoculation-Malaria," 211–12.

72. Bruetsch and Bahr, 221.

73. Bruetsch, "The Histopathology of Therapeutic (Tertian) Malaria."

74. Bruetsch, "Why Malaria Cures General Paralysis," 216.

75. CSH annual report, 1934, ISA.

76. CSH annual report, 1930, 27, ISA.

77. CSH annual report, 1932, 23, ISA.

78. Bruetsch, "Penicillin or Malaria Therapy in the Treatment of General Paralysis?," 368.

79. Cowan, *A Social History of American Technology*, 310–17.

80. Bud, *Penicillin*, 59.

81. Bruetsch, "Malaria Therapy in Syphilitic Primary Optic Atrophy," 16.

82. "Bruetsch Research Notes: Indications and Contraindications for Malarial Therapy," CSH, Walter L. Bruetsch files, box 9, folder 10.

83. Bruetsch, "Why Malaria Cures General Paralysis," 213, 215.
84. Bahr, "My Fifty Years of Psychiatry," 511.
85. Bahr, 511.

Chapter 3. Supplying the Research

1. Henry Boston is a pseudonym. All patient names—with the exception of Mabel Smith—have been changed in order to protect patient privacy. Patient file #17560, Central State Hospital (CSH) patient records, Indiana State Archives (ISA).
2. Rydell and Schiavo, *Designing Tomorrow*, 1–21.
3. Mabel Smith patient file, CSH patient records.
4. See, e.g., Fox and Swazey, *The Courage to Fail*; Halpern, *Lesser Harms*, 7–8.
5. Bruetsch's results aligned with those of other malaria therapy researchers nationally and internationally at the time. See chapter 2.
6. Brandt, *No Magic Bullet*.
7. Susan M. Reverby discusses the importance of highlighting the voices of those who suffered; see Reverby, "Suffering and Resistance, Voice and Agency," 270.
8. Crenner, "The Tuskegee Syphilis Study," 256; According to Suzanne Poirier, "about one-third of untreated patients develop tertiary syphilis," of which a smaller portion includes neurosyphilis. Poirier, *Chicago's War on Syphilis, 1937–1940*, 3.
9. Several patient files note that changes in a loved one's behavior began a year or more prior to their admission to CSH, gradually worsening over time. See, e.g., patient files #12794, #14360, #16313, #18033, CSH patient records.
10. It is important to note that not all illnesses necessarily lead to disability. See Nielsen, *A Disability History of the United States*, xiv.
11. On the difficulty of understanding another person's experience of pain, see Fuller, *The Body of Faith*, 105–7.
12. Both City Hospital and the county jails were often used to "restrain" those suffering from neurosyphilis until a space at CSH could be acquired. See, e.g., patient file #17344, CSH patient records.
13. Patient file #17560, CSH patient records.
14. County jails in particular were ill-quipped to handle the care of those suffering from general paresis. See patient file #16378, CSH patient records. Although City Hospital was also not equipped for long-term neurosyphilis care, it began administering malaria therapy at some point. Some patients are noted as having been treated with malaria at City Hospital prior to admission at CSH.
15. Patient file #16378, CSH patient records.
16. Patient files #12794, #16313, CSH patient records.
17. These accounts come from, respectively, patient files #14627, #14279, #16495, #15591, #20619, #16669, #15741, CSH patient records.

18. For more on vicarious shame, see Sedgwick and Frank, *Shame and Its Sisters*, 160.

19. Patient file #18275, CSH patient records.

20. Patient files #17053, #14987, #14963, CSH patient records.

21. On experiencing shame due to another's "shamelessness," see Sedgwick and Frank, *Shame and Its Sisters*, 160.

22. Patient files #16425, #16540, CSH patient records.

23. Patient files #17933, #14711, #16904, CSH patient records.

24. *Schloendorff v. Society of New York Hospital*, 211 N.Y. 125 (N.Y. 1914), quoted in Bazzano, Durant, and Brantley, "A Modern History of Informed Consent," 82.

25. Halpern, *Lesser Harms*, 3–4.

26. Gambino, "Fevered Decisions," 45; see also Baker, *Anglo-American Medical Ethics and Medical Jurisprudence*; Cooper, "Trial by Accident"; Fox and Swazey, *The Courage to Fail*; Halpern, *Lesser Harms*; Lederer, *Subjected to Science*.

27. Eldridge et al., "Treatment of Paresis," 1097; Gambino, "Fevered Decisions"; Lederer, *Subjected to Science*.

28. Matthew Gambino distinguishes between "clinical and research ethics," suggesting that because consent was given for treatment, ethical "transgressions" occurred less often on the research side of the malaria therapy experiment, and more often in its "clinical" practice. See Gambino, "Fevered Decisions," 45.

29. CSH annual report, 1937, 20, ISA.

30. Zwicker, "Experimenting with Radium Therapy," 194.

31. As Sydney A. Halpern notes, the "rules of consent were contingent upon both the status of the subject and the expected outcome of the intervention." Halpern, *Lesser Harms*, 4.

32. Halpern, *Lesser Harms*, 4. Susan Burch explains ableism as a "system of power and privilege that hierarchically organizes people and societies based on particular cultural values of productivity, competitive achievement, efficiency, capacity, and progress." Burch, *Committed*, 9.

33. Halpern, *Lesser Harms*, 4, 7–8; see also Fox and Swazey, *The Courage to Fail*; Scull, *Desperate Remedies*.

34. Many patient files at CSH include autopsy consent forms or copies of requests for such, but neither standard consent forms regarding treatment nor requests for such were found. CSH annual reports from the 1920s and 1930s and other archival records also do not include any mention of consent for treatment.

35. Wolfgang U. Eckart calls this disregard the "dark side of human experiment." Eckart, *Man, Medicine, and the State*, 9.

36. CSH, Walter L. Bruetsch files, box 2, folder 7, Indiana State Archives; Bruetsch, "Why Malaria Cures General Paralysis."

37. CSH annual report, 1937, 23–24, ISA; CSH annual report, 1941, 13, ISA.

38. CSH annual report, 1941, 27, ISA.

39. Bruetsch, "Penicillin or Malaria Therapy in the Treatment of General Paralysis?," 368.

40. Ben-Moshe, "Disabling Incarceration," 385; see also Burch, *Committed*, 16.

41. Imada, "Family History as Disability History," 2.

42. Patient files #13323, #13856, CSH patient records.

43. Patient files #16526, #17933, #16962, CSH patient records.

44. Elaine Scarry, quoted in Fuller, *The Body of Faith*, 107.

45. Patient file #16749, CSH patient records.

46. This is not a perfect comparison, given that Braslow's study and my own employ different methodological approaches and different datasets. For instance, Braslow analyzed a random sampling of files at a California institution, whereas I look exclusively at the files of those who died at CSH. See Braslow, "The Influence of a Biological Therapy on Physicians' Narratives and Interrogations"; Braslow, *Mental Ills and Bodily Cures*, 71.

47. Patient file #17078, CSH patient records.

48. Patient file #17078, CSH patient records.

49. Patient files #16526, #14627, CSH patient records.

50. Patient files #16744, #17344, CSH patient records.

51. See, e.g., "Help Shortage Cited in Killing," *Indianapolis Times*, August 8, 1945, 9; "Find Woman Dead, Jammed into Closet," *Indianapolis Times*, October 31, 1929, 1; "Inmate Death Brings Plans for Shakeup," *Indianapolis Times*, August 1, 1938, 1; "Wilson Ends Probe of Inmate's Death," *Indianapolis Times*, August 1938, 3, 8; all accessed through Indiana State Library (ISL).

52. CSH annual report, 1924, 39, ISA.

53. CSH annual report, 1926, 43, ISA.

54. CSH annual report, 1927, 46, ISA.

55. CSH annual report, 1930, 20, ISA.

56. CSH annual report, 1930, 20.

57. CSH annual report, 1929, 21, ISA.

58. Patient file #17933, CSH patient records.

59. "Inmate Death Brings Plans for Shakeup," *Indianapolis Times*, August 1, 1938, 1, ISL. No mention of the scalding was made in the 1938 CSH annual report.

60. CSH annual report, 1926, 43, ISA.

61. "State Orders Insane Moved," *Indianapolis Times*, November 2, 1927, 4, ISL.

62. In the 1924 annual report, Bahr quoted from over thirty years of reports that had repeatedly attempted to call attention to the "appalling," "horrific," "deplorable" conditions of the building known as the "Department for Men." See CSH annual report, 1924, 34–36, ISA.

63. Patient files #17396, #16936, CSH patient records.

64. By 1932, the heading "Escapes" is mostly absent from the annual reports, as are specific numbers of escapees. Instead, the 1933 annual report

merely notes that there were "few escapes." See CSH annual reports, 1924–32, ISA.

65. Ben-Moshe, "Disabling Incarceration," 385; Burch, *Committed*, 16.

66. "Find Woman Dead, Jammed into Closet," *Indianapolis Times*, October 31, 1929, 1, ISL.

67. In one example, the patient's file included a discharge date that was after the death date; see patient file #15649, CSH patient records. By 1932 annual reports stopped including tallies of escapes.

68. Edith Sutton is a pseudonym. Patient file #15649, CSH patient records.

69. Patient file #15649, CSH patient records.

70. Patient file #18019, CSH patient records. Notably, religious beliefs appear to have not prevented malaria treatment in this case, only the administration of other medications.

71. See Rembis, *Writing Mad Lives in the Age of the Asylum*.

72. CSH annual reports, 1927, 25; 1931, 22–23; 1946, 22; all in ISA.

73. This latter suggestion is corroborated by other historians' work. See Braslow, *Mental Ills and Bodily Cures*; Humphreys, "Whose Body? Which Disease?"; Reverby, *Examining Tuskegee*, 163.

74. Patient file #18275, CSH patient records.

75. Patient files #18019, #19007, CSH patient records.

76. See, e.g., Lombardo, *A Century of Eugenics in America*; Rembis, *Defining Deviance*; A. M. Stern, *Eugenic Nation*.

77. Patient file #17637, CSH patient records.

78. Patient files #14360, #16441, #18019, #18338, #19007, CSH patient records.

79. CSH annual report, 1926, 24, ISA.

80. CSH annual report, 1926, 24, ISA.

81. CSH annual report, 1927, 27, ISA.

82. CSH annual report, 1929, 38, ISA.

83. See, e.g., patient file #13886, CSH patient records.

84. Patient file #17356, CSH patient records.

85. Patient file #16431, CSH patient records.

86. That said, Superintendent Bahr later reported on one member of this group who suffered from typhoid fever, noting that the patient's physical recovery had been similar to those treated with malaria therapy. CSH annual report, 1929, 36, ISA.

87. Patient file #17743, CSH patient records.

88. Patient file #17960, CSH patient records.

89. CSH annual report, 1928, 36, ISA.

90. Patient file #16167, CSH patient records.

91. It should be noted here that some of those deemed cured may have relapsed years later. For statistics, see CSH annual report, 1928, 28, ISA.

92. Davis, *The Cruel Madness of Love*, 188.

93. Patient file #16936, CSH patient records; see also, e.g., patient file #17680.

94. Patient file #17828, CSH patient records.
95. Patient files #18033, #16850, CSH patient records.
96. CSH annual report, 1926, 23, ISA.
97. Patient files #17168, #16572, #13242, CSH patient records.
98. Davis, *The Cruel Madness of Love*, 188.
99. Davis, 154.
100. Patient file #17180, CSH patient records; see also, e.g., patient file #17947.

Chapter 4. Race, Gender, and Neurosyphilis

1. Hazel Morrison lays out the ways that patient case notes do both: reflect and re-create. See Morrison, "Constructing Patient Stories," 84–85.
2. See, e.g., Christopher Crenner's detailed historical exploration of "racial nervous resistance" in the Tuskegee syphilis study: Crenner, "The Tuskegee Syphilis Study."
3. According to Paul A. Lombardo and Gregory M. Dorr, twentieth-century eugenics "reinforced and updated the 'racial medicine' of the nineteenth century, establishing it on firmly modern, scientific grounds." Lombardo and Dorr, "Eugenics, Medical Education, and the Public Health Service," 292.
4. Historian Erika Dyck writes, "although eugenics emerged as a transnational ideology, its expression was more regional in character." Dyck, *Facing Eugenics*, 7.
5. See Jones, *Bad Blood*; Reverby, *Examining Tuskegee*.
6. As scholars Karen E. Fields and Barbara J. Fields observe, Thomas Jefferson's *Notes on the State of Virginia* (1785) is filled with scientific racism. See Fields and Fields, *Racecraft*, 18; see also Hunt-Kennedy, *Between Fitness and Death*; Sussman, *The Myth of Race*; Washington, *Medical Apartheid*; Yudell, *Race Unmasked*.
7. Humphreys, *Malaria*, 57, 59–60; Parsons, *From Asylum to Prison*, 14.
8. Sussman, *The Myth of Race: The Troubling Persistence of an Unscientific Idea*, (Cambridge, MA: Harvard University Press, 2014), 43–63.
9. Lombardo and Dorr, "Eugenics, Medical Education, and the Public Health Service," 293. See also Yudell, *Race Unmasked*.
10. Historian Christopher Crenner writes about the "neurosyphilis paradox," a concept he explains as "the notion that a racially prevalent disease had a racially rare complication." Crenner, "The Tuskegee Syphilis Study," 251, and see 249. See also Lombardo, *Three Generations, No Imbeciles*; Lombardo and Dorr, "Eugenics, Medical Education, and the Public Health Service." Thomas Parran, US surgeon general in the 1930s, repeated this erroneous belief in his 1937 book about syphilis; see Parran, *Shadow on the Land*.
11. Crenner, "The Tuskegee Syphilis Study," 252–53.
12. Summers, "Suitable Care of the African When Afflicted with Insanity," 67–68.

13. Crenner, "The Tuskegee Syphilis Study," 253; Gambino, "Fevered Decisions," 41; see also Reverby, *Examining Tuskegee*, 160–63.

14. Jonathan M. Metzl explains that "race impacts medical communication because racial tensions are structured into clinical interactions long before doctors or patients enter examination rooms.... Anxieties about racial difference shape diagnostic criteria, health-care policies, medical and popular attitudes about mentally ill persons, the structures of treatment facilities, and, ultimately, the conversations that take place there within." Metzl, *The Protest Psychosis*, xi.

15. As Keith Wailoo argues in his historical study of sickle cell anemia, "the ways in which diseases are defined, characterized, and dramatized provide a window on social relations and social values." See Wailoo, *Dying in the City of the Blues*, 2.

16. Sample, "A Truly Midwestern City," 130.

17. In his 1927 report for the Indianapolis Foundation, Dr. William H. Walsh noted that the university system of hospitals as well as most religiously affiliated hospitals refused Black patients. At Saint Vincent Hospital, for example, the mother superior acknowledged that at one time they had taken in "colored patients," but white people had "made such a fuss" that it became unsustainable. Walsh, "Report of a Study of the Hospital Accommodations for Colored People in Indianapolis," 7, Indianapolis Foundation Records (IFR), box 60, file 37, University Library Special Collections and Archives, Indianapolis University–Purdue University Indianapolis.

18. Moore, *Citizen Klansmen*, 64.

19. As Linda Gordon has written of its pervasive influence, the Klan seemed "ordinary and respectable to its contemporaries." Gordon, *The Second Coming of the KKK*, 3.

20. Walsh, "Report of a Study of the Hospital Accommodations for Colored People in Indianapolis," 3.

21. Walsh, 8.

22. Anne E. Parsons notes that state mental institutions served primarily "white and middle-aged" people; Parsons, *From Asylum to Prison*, 5. Records from CSH are unclear about whether patients were racially segregated. Nicole R. Kobrowski notes that in 1856, the CSH superintendent argued that Black patients should be admitted, but said that it was "absolutely necessary to build rooms isolated and purposely for them." Unattributed quote in Kobrowski, *Fractured Intentions*, 30. There is no mention in the patient records or institutional files from the 1920s–1940s of racially segregated spaces, but that does not preclude the possibility of a practice of racially segregating patients.

23. Patient files #16495, #16850, #18193, #16702, #17089, CSH patient records, Indiana State Archives (ISA).

24. As scholars Karen E. Fields and Barbara J. Fields note, such historical conclusions, based as they were on stereotypes and "folk thought," do not

make "genetic" or scientific sense. See Fields and Fields, *Racecraft*, 5–6, 8–9, 16–19, 41, 50–57. See also Yudell, *Race Unmasked*, 4.

25. Summers, "Suitable Care of the African When Afflicted with Insanity," 74.

26. For instance, one such patient who was suspected by the medical examiner of having "syphilis of the nervous system" appears to have nonetheless gone untreated without any further explanation. See patient file #18409, CSH patient records.

27. Bahr, "The So-Called Recovery of Paresis," CSH, Walter L. Bruetsch files, box 2, folder 7, ISA.

28. See, e.g., patient files #16441, #16850, CSH patient records.

29. Margaret Humphreys details the history of shifting medical beliefs about race and malaria. See Humphreys, *Malaria*, 14–20, 57–68. CSH claims appear to slightly predate the "revived" discussion that Humphreys outlines.

30. Humphreys notes that Boyd was a malaria researcher rather than a neurosyphilis researcher. See Humphreys, "Whose Body? Which Disease?," 64; Humphreys, *Malaria*, 66.

31. Additionally, Bruetsch and Bahr observed that two Black patients they inoculated with malaria did not spike high fevers, but nonetheless demonstrated significant improvement; they used this observation to buttress their developing medical claim that it wasn't just the fever, but the malaria itself that cured neurosyphilis. See CSH annual report, 1929, 33, ISA.

32. Reverby, *Examining Tuskegee*, 161–62.

33. Susan M. Reverby points out the irony in these two roles. Reverby, 163.

34. Reverby writes, "despite his education and authority, Dibble, as with every other African American in the country, dealt daily with the culture of humiliation that sought to keep whites in power." She explains that Dr. Dibble was a "race and science man," committed to both racial uplift and scientific advancement. Reverby, *Examining Tuskegee*, 154, 160, and see 152–66.

35. One exception is noted in the 1929 annual report. One Black man suffering from neurosyphilis was inoculated *five* times at CSH in the span of just four months. This man was indeed reported as cured and discharged. See CSH annual report, 1929, 33, ISA.

36. Patient file #17798, CSH patient records.

37. Quoted in Reverby, *Examining Tuskegee*, 162.

38. Humphreys, *Malaria*, 66. For more on the extreme dangers of the *P. falciparum* strain and the ethical issues this posed, see Humphreys, "Whose Body? Which Disease?," 70–71.

39. CSH annual report, 1940, 21, ISA.

40. Patient file #20619, CSH patient records.

41. For more on the history of medical researchers' race-based observations as well as the concept of acquired immunity, see Humphreys, *Malaria*, 61–68.

42. Explaining racecraft, Fields and Fields write, "the action and imagining are collective yet individual, day-to-day yet historical, and consequential

even though nested in mundane routine." See Fields and Fields, *Racecraft*, 5, 18–19.

43. Such constructions of race occurred at institutions beyond CSH. For instance, in his study of malaria therapy treatment at Saint Elizabeths, Matthew Gambino concludes that it "represents both a case study in the history of racialized medicine and a challenge to what we might expect such an episode to look like." Gambino, "Fevered Decisions," 46.

44. In his history of sickle cell anemia, Wailoo notes the development of theories in the 1950s that suggested "that the sickle cell trait began as a beneficial evolutionary protection against malaria." People with the trait were not ill and were supposedly "well adapted to survive in malarial surroundings," but it was believed that if two parents passed the trait to a child, this "double-dose" caused illness. See Wailoo, *Dying in the City of the Blues*, 6. Kenyan researcher Anthony C. Allison, who first proffered this theory in 1954, cited by Wailoo, specifically mentions the malarial treatment of syphilis as an initial point of connection for sickle cell researchers. See Wailoo, 236n10; see also Allison, "The Discovery of Resistance to Malaria of Sickle-Cell Heterozygotes," 280; Humphreys, *Malaria*, 66–68.

45. Fields and Fields, *Racecraft*, 18–19; for more on the history of race in science, see Yudell, *Race Unmasked*.

46. As Parsons notes, gender segregation constituted an intentional effort to restrict patients' reproductive abilities. See Parsons, *From Asylum to Prison*, 14. Erin Gallagher-Cohoon has argued that a US Public Health Service syphilis experiment conducted in Guatemala in 1946, which also used gender segregation, erroneously assumed heterosexuality. See Gallagher-Cohoon, "Despite Being 'Known, Highly Promiscuous, and Active.'"

47. See, e.g., patient files #12794, #14627, #16441, #17396, CSH patient records.

48. Patient file #16441, CSH patient records.

49. See, e.g., Rembis, *Defining Deviance*; A. M. Stern, *Eugenic Nation*.

50. Patient files #18142, #16431, #17669, CSH patient records.

51. Patient file #16441, CSH patient records.

52. Lunbeck, *The Psychiatric Persuasion*, 50–54.

53. Patient file #16892, CSH patient records; and see patient file #14156.

54. Patient files #14963, #16744, CSH patient records.

55. See, e.g., patient file #16310, CSH patient records.

56. Lunbeck, *The Psychiatric Persuasion*.

57. Patient files #14627, #14861, CSH patient records.

58. CSH annual report, 1927, 18, ISA.

59. CSH annual report, 1931, 24, ISA.

60. CSH annual report, 1941, 21, ISA.

61. CSH annual report, 1941, 20, ISA.

62. Metzl argues that "the rhetorics of health and illness become effective ways of policing the boundaries of civil society." Metzl, *The Protest Psychosis*, xxi.

63. Renée C. Fox and Judith P. Swazey explore quality-of-life issues for kidney transplant patients, whose lives were extended by medical technologies. See Fox and Swazey, *The Courage to Fail*, 378.

64. Patient file #14963, CSH patient records.

65. Mabel Smith patient file, CSH patient records.

66. Dyck, *Facing Eugenics*; Lombardo, *Three Generations, No Imbeciles*, 24. See also Whitaker, *Mad in America*, 41–73; and for more on the history of sterilization, see Reilly, *The Surgical Solution*.

67. "Bruetsch Research Notes: Indications and Contraindications for Malarial Therapy," 12–13, CSH, Walter L. Bruetsch files, box 9, folder 10.

68. "Bruetsch Research Notes," 13.

69. "Bruetsch Research Notes," 12.

70. Patient file #16640, CSH patient records.

71. Lantzer, "The Indiana Way of Eugenics," 37.

72. For more on the institutionalization of eugenics, see Rembis, *Defining Deviance*, 26–28.

73. A. M. Stern, "From Legislation to Lived Experience," 99, 106.

74. CSH annual reports divided women's surgeries into two categories: hysterectomies (uterus removal) and salpingectomies (fallopian tube removal). Of the twenty-seven sterilizing surgeries performed between 1935 and 1938, thirteen were hysterectomies and fourteen were salpingectomies. See CSH annual reports, 1935–38, ISA.

75. Patient file #18490, CSH patient records.

76. For more on the connection between social reformers, modern medicine, and eugenics, see Lombardo, *Three Generations, No Imbeciles*; Lombardo and Dorr, "Eugenics, Medical Education, and the Public Health Service"; A. M. Stern, *Eugenic Nation*; Sussman, *The Myth of Race*, 43–63.

77. Lombardo, *Three Generations, No Imbeciles*, 46. For early examples of eugenics-inspired restrictive marriage laws, see Reilly, *The Surgical Solution*, 26–27.

78. Patient files #18019, #19007, CSH patient records.

79. Mabel Smith patient file, CSH patient records.

80. A. M. Stern, "From Legislation to Lived Experience," 104–6.

Chapter 5. Dying from Neurosyphilis and the Silencing of Disability

1. Mabel Smith patient file, Central State Hospital (CSH) patient records, Indiana State Archives (ISA). Mabel Smith, certificate of death, Marion County (IN) Health Department, filed March 1, 1931 (in author's possession).

2. For a description of "vicarious" shame, see Sedgwick and Frank, *Shame and Its Sisters*, 160.

3. Bahr, "Nervous and Mental Diseases in Relation to Public Health," 7.

4. Fink, *All Our Families*, ix–xix, 18.

5. Ariès, *The Hour of Our Death*, 409–74, 559, 561, 563–71, 611–14.

6. As Gary Laderman puts it, the very "successes of medicine began to transform death into something shameful and unnatural." Laderman, *The Sacred Remains*, 7.

7. Nicole R. Kobrowski notes the "confusion" surrounding patient burial at the institution. Patients buried prior to 1905 were not clearly or systematically documented, and in the years after 1905, several parcels of land on-site served as burial sites. The 1995 effort involved relabeling markers for individuals known to have been buried on-site. More recently, according to Kobrowski, volunteers at the Indiana Medical History Museum have worked to create a more accurate and updated cemetery listing. Kobrowski, *Fractured Intentions*, 180–81. Museum director Sarah Halter noted that this work was still in process as of May 2023 (pers. comm.). In November 2020 construction at the behest of the Indianapolis Metropolitan Police Department to build a new K-9 training facility near the CSH cemetery resulted in the disruption and "mangling" of the remains of three people buried there. The Indiana Medical History Museum released a statement, noting, "We may never know the extent of this potential damage. . . . This is simply not OK." See Andrea, "Human Remains at Central State 'Mangled.'"

8. CSH annual reports, 1924–40, ISA.

9. CSH continued to admit significantly higher numbers of patients suffering from syphilis infection than did state mental institutions across the country, well into the 1930s. The 1938 percentage of new admissions was 24 percent. See CSH annual report, 1938, ISA.

10. "Autopsies for Curiosity Laid to Coroner," *Indianapolis Times*, November 19, 1931, 1, Indiana State Library (ISL). Meanwhile, the pressure to secure cadavers for medical training continued. A 1927 Indiana law required that anyone practicing medicine or surgery must have at least two years of "premedic" work "in an institution where instruction includes dissection of the human body." See "Chiropractors Seek New Law," *Indianapolis Times*, October 24, 1933, 5, ISL.

11. Drew Gilpin Faust discusses the "fundamental uncertainty of the boundary between life and death." Faust, *This Republic of Suffering*, 75–76. Ariès also examines this "unclear boundary between life and death." Ariès, *The Hour of Our Death*, 396.

12. Halperin, "A Glimpse of Our Past"; Humphrey, "Dissection and Discrimination"; Laderman, *The Sacred Remains*, 78; Tuggle, *The Afterlives of Specimens*, 6.

13. Faust argues that although embalming was introduced prior to the war, it was primarily only used for preserving bodies for dissection, and that the war itself is what created the shift toward the widespread practice of embalming. See Faust, *This Republic of Suffering*, 61–101. Lindsey Tuggle notes that in the wake of his assassination, President Abraham Lincoln was embalmed. She also argues that the transcendental poet Walt Whitman symbolized the

growing acceptance of dissection as he himself transitioned from an initial opposition to dissection, requesting that his body be autopsied and his brain studied by science. See Tuggle, *The Afterlives of Specimens*, 1–23, esp. 6–10 and 22; see also Laderman, *The Sacred Remains*, esp. 96–102.

14. Shultz, *Body Snatching*, 14.

15. Humphrey, "Dissection and Discrimination," 821; Laderman, *The Sacred Remains*, 73–85; Shultz, *Body Snatching*, 14; Goodwin, *Black Markets*, 172–73.

16. *Resurrectionist* was a term used for grave robbers. As Harriet A. Washington notes, "Black graveyards were the favored hunting grounds of northern body snatchers." Washington, *Medical Apartheid*, 131. See also Goodwin, *Black Markets*, 171–75.

17. Blakely and Harrington, *Bones in the Basement*.

18. Tuggle, *The Afterlives of Specimens*, 30–36; Goodwin, *Black Markets*, 171–75.

19. Halperin, "A Glimpse of Our Past." As David C. Humphrey wrote in 1973, "the anatomy laws confined dissections to a voiceless, widely-scorned segment of society." Humphrey, "Dissection and Discrimination," 824; see also Tuggle, *The Afterlives of Specimens*, 6.

20. Halperin, "A Glimpse of Our Past," 491.

21. For examples of grave robbing reported in the local press, see "Body Snatching," *Indianapolis Journal*, December 8, 1873, 1, ISL; "The Cause of Science," *Bloomington Progress*, November 6, 1872, 1, ISL; "Charles Hemmerle, a German . . . ," *Indianapolis News*, December 30, 1875, 2, ISL; "Resurrection and Dissection," *Indianapolis News*, February 25, 1879, 3, ISL.

22. "Resurrection and Dissection," *Indianapolis News*, February 25, 1879, 3, ISL. See also Washington, *Medical Apartheid*.

23. Humphrey, "Dissection and Discrimination," 824.

24. Beckley, "King of Ghouls."

25. Humphrey, "Dissection and Discrimination," 824.

26. "Autopsies for Curiosity Laid to Coroner," *Indianapolis Times*, November 19, 1931, 1, ISL.

27. Vehling was later convicted in a jury trial for soliciting a bribe and sentenced to six years in prison. He tried to appeal the sentencing based on his opinion that one jury member was "insane." See "Vehling to Have Court Hearing Monday on Coram Nobis Writ," *Indianapolis Times*, March 20, 1937, 4, ISL.

28. Laderman argues that medical schools were "obsessed with the dead." Laderman, *The Sacred Remains*, 83–85.

29. CSH annual report, 1940, 25, ISA.

30. CSH annual report, 1939, 27, ISA.

31. See CSH annual reports, 1924–45, ISA.

32. See CSH annual reports, 1924–45, ISA.

33. CSH annual report, 1930, 34, ISA.

34. Kobrowski notes that autopsy viewing was moved to Methodist Hospital in the 1960s. See Kobrowski, *Fractured Intentions*, 98.

35. CSH annual report, 1938, 38, ISA.

36. "Chiropractors Seek New Law," *Indianapolis Times*, October 24, 1933, 5, ISL.

37. Nystrom, "The Bioarchaeology of Structural Violence and Dissection," 769.

38. CSH annual report, 1941, 25, ISA; CSH annual report, 1948, 27, ISA.

39. Patient file #16669, CSH patient records.

40. Washington, *Medical Apartheid*, 134.

41. Washington, 134–35; Scott, "Woman Sues over Display." For a longer history of racism in medical training at the Medical College of Georgia, see Blakely and Harrington, *Bones in the Basement*.

42. CSH annual reports, 1924–40, ISA. The years 1932 and 1933 recorded unusually low rates of autopsy, coming in at just 13.2 percent and 18.3 percent of total deaths, respectively. The annual reports for these years include explanatory notes regarding these low numbers, with promises to return to the higher rate of autopsy in succeeding years.

43. Patient file #17344, CSH patient records.

44. Patient file #18275, CSH patient records.

45. Patient files #18275, #16640, CSH patient records.

46. Patient file #11797, CSH patient records.

47. In one pathology report Dr. Bruetsch concluded that "from the gros [sic] aspect of the brain a diagnosis of G.P. could not be made." Patient file #16572, CSH patient records.

48. Patient file #18242, CSH patient records.

49. Patient file #16425, CSH patient records.

50. Patient files #17929, #18275, CSH patient records. Another patient was autopsied within ninety minutes of death; see patient file #18033.

51. Faust, *This Republic of Suffering*, 396.

52. Laderman, *The Sacred Remains*, 31.

53. CSH annual report, 1931, 35, ISA.

54. Bruetsch's pathology reports were quite extensive; occasionally patient files included autopsy notes written by doctors other than Bruetsch, but his notes are primary. Examples of Bruetsch's lengthy autopsy reports include patient files #15905, #17029, #18271, CSH patient records.

55. Washington, *Medical Apartheid*, 132; "Resurrection and Dissection," *Indianapolis News*, February 25, 1879, 3, ISL.

56. As Suzanne M. Shultz notes, although "religious objections are often cited as the primary reason for denying the use of human cadavers for the study of anatomy by dissection/autopsy, there are no specific Catholic or Protestant prohibitions against the practice." Shultz, *Body Snatching*, 7.

57. Scholar Jenny Reardon discusses modern efforts to define "rights" in a way that might encourage bodily donations that benefit "humanity." See Reardon, *The Postgenomic Condition*, 12–13.

58. Autopsy records reveal that some patients' brains and other tissues were dissected more than once, sometimes several months or years after the first dissection. See, e.g., patient file #17089, CSH patient records.

59. Ariès, *The Hour of Our Death*, 612.

60. Ariès, 612–13.

Conclusion

1. Walter L. Bruetsch to Dr. Thomas B. Turner, May 12, 1958, Thomas B. Turner collection, box 4, folder 2.02.087, Alan Mason Chesney Medical Archives, Johns Hopkins University and Medicine.

2. Thomas B. Turner to Dr. Walter L. Bruetsch, July 14, 1958, Thomas B. Turner collection, box 4, folder 2.02.087.

3. Reprint of Bruetsch, "The Collagen Diseases," Thomas B. Turner collection, box 52, folder 8.2.1.08.003.

4. Marks, *The Progress of Experiment*, 28.

5. Stearns, *Shame*, 8.

6. Excerpted in Sedgwick and Frank, *Shame and Its Sisters*, 153.

7. For more on the history of shame and honor culture, see Stearns, *Shame*, 59, 74–76. For more on the persistence of shame associated with women's sexuality and reproduction, see Adams, *Enduring Shame*, 4.

8. Cemetery records note that Irvin Ward was buried in the same plot as Mabel Smith, and yet only a headstone with her name exists at the site. Information based on telephone conversation, official records, and visit to the Holy Cross and Saint Joseph Cemetery in Indianapolis, May 2016.

9. See, e.g., Fink, *All Our Families*. For a related discussion of how historical silences reproduce racism, see Trouillot, *Silencing the Past*, 26.

Bibliography

Archival Collections

Autopsy Reports. Indiana Medical History Museum, Indianapolis.
Central State Hospital (CHS), Annual Reports, 1923–49. Indiana State Archives (ISA), Indianapolis.
Central State Hospital (CHS), Correspondence. Indiana State Archives (ISA), Indianapolis.
Central State Hospital (CHS), Patient Records. Indiana State Archives (ISA), Indianapolis.
Central State Hospital, Walter L. Bruetsch files. Indiana State Archives (ISA), Indianapolis.
City Hospital, Admission Books. Indiana Historical Society, Indianapolis.
Indianapolis Foundation Records (IFR), 1916–2000. University Library Special Collections and Archives, Indiana University–Purdue University Indianapolis.
Marion County Naturalizations. Digital Collection, Indiana State Archives (ISA), Indianapolis.
Newspaper holdings (online and print). Indiana State Library (ISL), Indianapolis.
St. John the Evangelist Catholic Church Archives, Baptism Registers. Indianapolis, IN.
St. John the Evangelist Catholic Church Archives, Marriage Registers. Indianapolis, IN.
Thomas B. Turner collection. Alan Mason Chesney Medical Archives. Johns Hopkins University and Medicine, Baltimore, MD.

Primary Sources and Manuscripts

Agnew, Anna. *From under the Cloud, or Personal Reminiscences of Insanity*. Cincinnati, OH: Robert Clarke, 1886.

Allison, Anthony C. "The Discovery of Resistance to Malaria of Sickle-Cell Heterozygotes." *Biochemistry and Molecular Biology Education* 30, no. 5 (2002): 279–87.

Bahr, Max. "Nervous and Mental Diseases in Relation to Public Health." Paper presented at the Indiana Health Conference and Health Officers School, Indianapolis, May 22–23, 1917.

Bahr, Max. "My Fifty Years of Psychiatry." *Journal of the Indiana State Medical Association* 45, no. 6 (1952): 510–13.

Bahr, Max. "The So-Called Recovery of Paresis." Paper presented for the Indianapolis Medical Society, November 18, 1930.

Bahr, Max, and W. L. Bruetsch. *Malaria Therapy of General Paresis and Allied Subjects.* Indianapolis, IN: Central State Hospital, 1940.

Bahr, Max, and W. L. Bruetsch. "Two Years' Experience with the Malarial Treatment of General Paralysis in a State Institution." *American Journal of Psychiatry* 84, no. 5 (1928): 715–27.

Bruetsch, Walter L. "The Collagen Diseases: Clues as to Their Etiology." *Transactions of the American Neurological Association* 94 (1969): 232–34.

Bruetsch, Walter L. "The Histopathology of Therapeutic (Tertian) Malaria." *American Journal of Psychiatry* 89, no. 1 (1932): 19–65.

Bruetsch, Walter L. "Julius Wagner-Jauregg, M.D.: Eminent Psychiatrist and Originator of the Malaria Treatment of Dementia Paralytica, 1857–1940." *Archives of Neurology and Psychiatry* 44, no. 6 (1940): 1319–22.

Bruetsch, Walter L. "Malaria Therapy in Syphilitic Primary Optic Atrophy." *Journal of the American Medical Association* 130, no. 1 (1946): 14–18.

Bruetsch, Walter L. "Max A. Bahr, M.D., 1874–1953." *American Journal of Psychiatry* 109, no. 10 (1953): 800.

Bruetsch, Walter L. "Penicillin or Malaria Therapy in the Treatment of General Paralysis? A Clinico-Anatomic Study." *Diseases of the Nervous System* 10, no. 12 (1949): 368–71.

Bruetsch, Walter L. "Why Malaria Cures General Paralysis." *Journal of the Indiana State Medical Association* 42, no. 3 (1949): 211–16.

Bruetsch, Walter L., and Max Bahr. "A Study of the Mechanism of Inoculation-Malaria on the Histopathologic Changes in Paresis." *Journal of Nervous and Mental Disease* 67, no. 3 (1928): 209–23.

Bunker, Henry A., Jr., and George H. Kirby. "Treatment of General Paralysis by Inoculation with Malaria: A First Report." *Journal of the American Medical Association* 84, no. 8 (1925): 563–68.

De Kruif, Paul. *Men against Death.* New York: Harcourt, Brace, 1932.

Eldridge, Watson W., John E. Lind, Samuel A. Silk, and P. J. Trentzsch. "Treatment of Paresis: Results of Inoculation with the Organism of Benign Tertian Malaria." *Journal of the American Medical Association* 84, no. 15 (1925): 1097–101.

Lewis, Nolan D. C., Lois D. Hubbard, and Edna G. Dyar. "The Malarial Treatment of Paretic Neurosyphilis." *American Journal of Psychiatry* 81, no. 2 (1924): 175–225.

Lies, Eugene T. *The Leisure of a People: A Report of a Recreation Survey of Indianapolis*. Indianapolis, IN: Council of Social Agencies and Indianapolis Foundation, 1929.

Lynd, Robert, and Helen Lynd. *Middletown: A Study in American Culture*. New York: Harcourt Brace, 1929.

Mental Defectives in Indiana: Third Report of the Indiana Committee on Mental Defectives to the Governor. Indianapolis, IN: W. B. Burford, 1922.

Merritt, Houston H., Raymond D. Adams, and Harry C. Solomon. *Neurosyphilis*. New York: Oxford University Press, 1946.

Moore, Joseph Earle. *The Modern Treatment of Syphilis*. 2nd ed. Springfield, IL: Charles C. Thomas, 1941.

New York Times. "One Malady Casts Out Another." July 7, 1925, 18.

O'Leary, Paul A. "Treatment of Neurosyphilis by Malaria: Report on the Three Years' Observation of the First One Hundred Patients Treated." *Journal of the American Medical Association* 89, no. 2 (1927): 95–100.

O'Leary, Paul A., William H. Goeckerman, and Stephen T. Parker. "Treatment of Neurosyphilis by Malaria: A Preliminary Report." *Archives of Dermatology and Syphilology* 13, no. 2 (1926): 301–20.

Parran, Thomas, Jr. *Shadow on the Land: Syphilis*. New York: Reynal and Hitchcock, 1937.

Scott, Jeffry. "Woman Sues over Display of Mom's Skeleton." *Atlanta Journal-Constitution*, March 16, 2003, A1.

Van Meter, F. J. "Malarial Treatment of General Paresis." *California and Western Medicine* 42, no. 5 (1934): 366–70.

Walsh, William H. "Report of a Study of the Hospital Accommodations for Colored People in Indianapolis." Study conducted under the auspices of the Indianapolis Foundation, IN, November 1927.

Secondary Sources

Adams, Heather Brook. *Enduring Shame: A Recent History of Unwed Pregnancy and Righteous Reproduction*. Charleston: University of South Carolina Press, 2022.

Andrea, Lawrence. "Human Remains at Central State 'Mangled' in IMPD Facility Construction, Museum Says." *Indianapolis Star*, November 24, 2020.

Appleman, Laura I. "Deviancy, Dependency, and Disability: The Forgotten History of Eugenics and Mass Incarceration." *Duke Law Journal* 68, no. 3 (2018): 418–78.

Ariès, Philippe. *The Hour of Our Death*. Translated by Helen Weaver. New York: Oxford University Press, 1981.

Bailey, Beth L. *From Front Porch to Back Seat: Courtship in Twentieth-Century America*. Baltimore, MD: Johns Hopkins University Press, 1989.

Baker, Robert, ed. *Anglo-American Medical Ethics and Medical Jurisprudence in the Nineteenth Century*. London: Kluwer Academic, 1995.

Bazzano, Lydia A., Jaquail Durant, and Paula Rhode Brantley. "A Modern History of Informed Consent and the Role of Key Information." *Ochsner Journal* 21, no. 1 (2021): 81–85.

Beckley, Lindsey. "'King of Ghouls,' Rufus Cantrell and Grave-Robbing in Indianapolis." *Untold Indiana* (blog). Indiana Historical Bureau, October 31, 2020. https://blog.history.in.gov/king-of-ghouls-rufus-cantrell-grave-robbing-in-indianapolis/.

Ben-Moshe, Liat. "Disabling Incarceration: Connecting Disability to Divergent Confinements in the USA." *Critical Sociology* 39, no. 3 (2011): 385–403.

Ben-Moshe, Liat, Chris Chapman, and Allison C. Carey, eds. *Disability Incarcerated: Imprisonment and Disability in the United States and Canada*. New York: Palgrave Macmillan, 2014.

Birzer, Bradley J. "Jean Baptiste Richardville: Miami Métis." In Edmunds, *Enduring Nations*, 94–108.

Blakely, Robert L., and Judith M. Harrington, eds. *Bones in the Basement: Postmortem Racism in Nineteenth-Century Medical Training*. Washington, DC: Smithsonian Institution Press, 1997.

Bonner, Thomas Neville. *American Doctors and German Universities: A Chapter in International Intellectual Relations, 1870–1914*. Lincoln: University of Nebraska Press, 1963.

Bonsett, Charles A. "Dr. Walter Bruetsch, Obituary." *Journal of the Indiana State Medical Association* 70, no. 3 (March 1977): 105.

Brandt, Allan M. *No Magic Bullet: A Social History of Venereal Disease in the United States since 1880*. New York: Oxford University Press, 1985.

Braslow, Joel. "The Influence of a Biological Therapy on Physicians' Narratives and Interrogations: The Case of General Paralysis of the Insane and Malaria Fever Therapy, 1910–1950." *Bulletin of the History of Medicine* 70, no. 4 (1996): 577–608.

Braslow, Joel. *Mental Ills and Bodily Cures: Psychiatric Treatment in the First Half of the Twentieth Century*. Berkeley: University of California Press, 1997.

Bristow, Nancy K. *Making Men Moral: Social Engineering during the Great War*. New York: New York University Press, 1996.

Buckles, Kacey, Melanie Guldi, and Joseph Price. "Changing the Price of Marriage: Evidence from Blood Test Requirements." *Journal of Human Resources* 46, no. 3 (2011): 539–67.

Bud, Robert. *Penicillin: Triumph and Tragedy*. New York: Oxford University Press, 2007.

Burch, Susan. *Committed: Remembering Native Kinship in and beyond Institutions*. Chapel Hill: University of North Carolina Press, 2021.

Burch, Susan. *Unspeakable: The Story of Junius Wilson*. Chapel Hill: University of North Carolina Press, 2007.

Burch, Susan, and Michael Rembis, eds. *Disability Histories*. Urbana: University of Illinois Press, 2014.

Cahn, Susan K. "Border Disorders: Mental Illness, Feminist Metaphor, and the Disordered Female Psyche in the Twentieth-Century United States." In Burch and Rembis, *Disability Histories*, 258–82.

Carlson, Elof Axel. "The Hoosier Connection: Compulsory Sterilization as Moral Hygiene." In Lombardo, *A Century of Eugenics in America*, 11–25.

Chapman, Chris, Allison C. Carey, and Liat Ben-Moshe. "Reconsidering Confinement: Interlocking Locations and Logics of Incarceration." In Ben-Moshe, Chapman, and Carey, *Disability Incarcerated*, 3–24.

Cooper, Melinda. "Trial by Accident: Tort Law, Industrial Risks, and the History of Medical Experiment." *Journal of Cultural Economy* 4, no. 1 (2011): 81–96.

Cowan, Ruth Schwartz. *A Social History of American Technology*. New York: Oxford University Press, 1997.

Crenner, Christopher. "The Tuskegee Syphilis Study and the Scientific Concept of Racial Nervous Resistance." *Journal of the History of Medicine and Allied Science* 67, no. 2 (2012): 244–80.

Davis, Gayle. *"The Cruel Madness of Love": Sex, Syphilis and Psychiatry in Scotland, 1880–1930*. New York: Rodopi, 2008.

D'Emilio, John, and Estelle B. Freedman. *Intimate Matters: A History of Sexuality in America*. 3rd ed. Chicago: University of Chicago Press, 2012.

Demos, John. "Shame and Guilt in Early New England." In *Emotion and Change: Toward a New Psychohistory*, edited by Carol Z. Stearns and Peter N. Stearns, 69–86. New York: Holmes and Meier, 1988.

Dittrich, Luke. *Patient H.M.: A Story of Memory, Madness, and Family Secrets*. New York: Random House, 2016.

Donaldson, Elizabeth J. "Revisiting the Corpus of the Madwoman: Further Notes toward a Feminist Disability Studies Theory of Mental Illness." In *Feminist Disability Studies*, edited by Kim Q. Hall, 91–114. Bloomington: Indiana University Press, 2011.

Dowling, Harry F. *Fighting Infection: Conquests of the Twentieth Century*. Cambridge, MA: Harvard University Press, 1977.

Dyck, Erika. *Facing Eugenics: Reproduction, Sterilization, and the Politics of Choice*. Toronto: University of Toronto Press, 2013.

Dyck, Erika, and Larry Stewart. Introduction to Dyck and Stewart, *The Uses of Humans in Experiment*, 1–27.

Dyck, Erika, and Larry Stewart, eds. *The Uses of Humans in Experiment: Perspectives from the 17th to the 20th Century*. Leiden: Brill Rodopi, 2016.

Eckart, Wolfgang U. *Man, Medicine, and the State: The Human Body as an Object of Government Sponsored Medical Research in the 20th Century*. Stuttgart: Steiner, 2006.

Edmunds, R. David, ed. *Enduring Nations: Native Americans in the Midwest*. Urbana: University of Illinois Press, 2008.

Edmunds, R. David. Introduction to Edmunds, *Enduring Nations*, 1–14.

Erevelles, Nirmalla. "Crippin' Jim Crow: Disability, Dis-Location, and the School-to-Prison Pipeline." In Ben-Moshe, Chapman, and Carey, *Disability Incarcerated*, 81–99.

Faust, Drew Gilpin. *This Republic of Suffering: Death and the American Civil War*. New York: Alfred A. Knopf, 2008.

Fields, Karen E., and Barbara J. Fields. *Racecraft: The Soul of Inequality in American Life*. London: Verso, 2012.

Fink, Jennifer Natalya. *All Our Families: Disability Lineage and the Future of Kinship*. Boston: Beacon Press, 2022.

Foucault, Michel. *History of Madness*. New York: Routledge, 2006.

Fox, Renée C., and Judith P. Swazey. *The Courage to Fail: A Social View of Organ Transplants and Dialysis*. London: Transaction, 2002.

Frank, Adam J., and Elizabeth A. Wilson. *A Silvan Tomkins Handbook: Foundations for Affect Theory*. Minneapolis: University of Minnesota Press, 2020.

Fuller, Robert C. *The Body of Faith: A Biological History of Religion in America*. Chicago: University of Chicago Press, 2013.

Gallagher-Cohoon, Erin. "Despite Being 'Known, Highly Promiscuous, and Active': Presumed Heterosexuality in the USPHS's STD Inoculation Study, 1946–48." *Canadian Bulletin of Medical History* 35, no. 2 (2018): 337–56.

Gambino, Matthew. "Fevered Decisions: Race, Ethics, and Clinical Vulnerability in the Malarial Treatment of Neurosyphilis, 1922–1953." *Hastings Center Report* 45, no. 4 (2015): 39–50.

Garland-Thomson, Rosemarie. "Feminist Disability Studies." *Signs* 30, no. 2 (2005): 1557–87.

Geller, Jeffrey L., and Maxine Harris, eds. *Women of the Asylum: Voices from behind the Walls, 1840–1945*. New York: Anchor Books, 1994.

Glass, James. "A Lesson in Indy's Transportation System." *Indianapolis Star*, February 3, 2019.

Goodwin, Michelle. *Black Markets: The Supply and Demand of Body Parts*. Cambridge: Cambridge University Press, 2006.

Gordon, Linda. *The Second Coming of the KKK: The Ku Klux Klan of the 1920s and the American Political Tradition*. New York: Liverwright, 2017.

Grob, Gerald. *The Inner World of American Psychiatry, 1890–1940: Selected Correspondence*. New Brunswick, NJ: Rutgers University Press, 1985.

Grob, Gerald. *The Mad among Us: A History of the Care of America's Mentally Ill*. New York: Free Press, 1994.

Halperin, Edward C. "A Glimpse of Our Past: The Poor, the Black, and the Marginalized as the Source of Cadavers in United States Anatomical Education." *Clinical Anatomy* 20, no. 5 (2007): 489–95.

Halpern, Sydney A. *Lesser Harms: The Morality of Risk in Medical Research*. Chicago: University of Chicago Press, 2004.

Helgeson, Jeffrey. "Politics in the Promised Land: How the Great Migration Shaped the American Midwest." In Lauck, Whitney, and Hogan, *Finding a New Midwestern History*, 111–26.

Hiro, Molly. "How It Feels to Be without a Face: Race and the Reorientation of Sympathy in the 1890s." *Novel: A Forum on Fiction* 39, no. 2 (2006): 179–203.

Horan, Rose Angela. *The Story of Old St. John's: A Parish Rooted in Pioneer Indianapolis*. Indianapolis, IN: Lithio Press, 1971.

Humphrey, David C. "Dissection and Discrimination: The Social Origins of Cadavers in America, 1760–1915." *Bulletin of New York Academic Medicine* 49, no. 9 (1973): 819–27.

Humphreys, Margaret. *Malaria: Poverty, Race, and Public Health in the United States*. Baltimore, MD: Johns Hopkins University Press, 2001.

Humphreys, Margaret. "Whose Body, Which Disease? Studying Malaria while Treating Neurosyphilis." In *Useful Bodies: Humans in the Service of Medical Science in the Twentieth Century*, edited by Jordan Goodman, Anthony McElligott, and Lara Marks, 53–77. Baltimore, MD: Johns Hopkins University Press, 2003.

Hunt-Kennedy, Stefanie. *Between Fitness and Death: Disability and Slavery in the Caribbean*. Chicago: University of Illinois Press, 2020.

Imada, Adria L. "Family History as Disability History: Native Hawaiians Surviving Medical Incarceration." *Disability Studies Quarterly* 41, no. 4 (2021). https://doi.org/10.18061/dsq.v41i4.8475.

Jacobson, Matthew Frye. *Roots Too: White Ethnic Revival in Post-Civil Rights America*. Cambridge, MA: Harvard University Press, 2006.

Jacobson, Matthew Frye. *Whiteness of a Different Color: European Immigrants and the Alchemy of Race*. Cambridge, MA: Harvard University Press, 1998.

Jensen, Kimberly. *Mobilizing Minerva: American Women in the First World War*. Urbana: University of Illinois Press, 2008.

Jones, James H. *Bad Blood: The Tuskegee Syphilis Experiment*. Boston: Free Press, 1993.

Kampmeier, Rudolph H. "Syphilis Therapy: An Historical Perspective." *Journal of the American Venereal Disease Association*. 3, no. 2 (1976): 99–108.

Kampmeier, Rudolph H. "Wagner von Jauregg and the Treatment of General Paresis by Fever." *Sexually Transmitted Diseases* 7, no. 3 (1980): 142–44.

King, Lucy Jane. *From under the Cloud at Seven Steeples: The Peculiarly Saddened Life of Anna Agnew at the Indiana Hospital for the Insane*. Zionsville, IN: Guild Press, 2002.

Kleinman, Arthur. *The Illness Narratives: Suffering, Healing, and the Human Condition*. New York: Basic Books, 1988.

Kline, Wendy. *Building a Better Race: Gender, Sexuality, and Eugenics from the Turn of the Century to the Baby Boom*. Berkeley: University of California Press, 2001.

Kobrowski, Nicole R. *Fractured Intentions: A History of Central State Hospital for the Insane*. Westfield, IN: Unseenpress.com, 2014.

Kudlick, Catherine. "Social History of Medicine and Disability History." In Rembis, Kudlick, and Nielsen, *The Oxford Handbook of Disability History*, 105–24.

Laderman, Gary. *The Sacred Remains: American Attitudes toward Death, 1799–1883*. New Haven, CT: Yale University Press, 1996.

Lantzer, Jason S. "The Indiana Way of Eugenics: Sterilization Laws, 1907–1974." In Lombardo, *A Century of Eugenics in America*, 26–45.

Lauck, Jon K., Joseph Hogan, and Gleaves Whitney. Introduction to Lauck, Whitney, and Hogan, *Finding a New Midwestern History*, xi–xxiii.

Lauck, Jon K., Gleaves Whitney, and Joseph Hogan, eds. *Finding a New Midwestern History*. Lincoln: University of Nebraska Press, 2018.

Leavitt, Judith Walzer. *Women and Health in America: Historical Readings*. Madison: University of Wisconsin Press, 1984.

Lederer, Susan E. *Subjected to Science: Human Experimentation in America before the Second World War*. Baltimore, MD: Johns Hopkins University Press, 1995.

Leon, Sharon M. *An Image of God: The Catholic Struggle with Eugenics*. Chicago: University of Chicago Press, 2013.

Lombardo, Paul A., ed. *A Century of Eugenics in America: From the Indiana Experiment to the Human Genome Era*. Bloomington: University of Indiana Press, 2011.

Lombardo, Paul A. *Three Generations, No Imbeciles: Eugenics, the Supreme Court, and Buck v. Bell*. Baltimore, MD: Johns Hopkins University Press, 2008.

Lombardo, Paul A., and Gregory M. Dorr. "Eugenics, Medical Education, and the Public Health Service: Another Perspective on the Tuskegee Syphilis Experiment." *Bulletin of the History of Medicine* 80, no. 2 (2006): 291–316.

Lunbeck, Elizabeth. *The Psychiatric Persuasion: Knowledge, Gender, and Power in Modern America*. Princeton, NJ: Princeton University Press, 1994.

MacLean, Nancy. *Behind the Mask of Chivalry: The Making of the Second Ku Klux Klan*. New York: Oxford University Press, 1994.

Marks, Harry M. *The Progress of Experiment: Science and Therapeutic Reform in the United States, 1900–1990*. New York: Cambridge University Press, 1997.

Metzl, Jonathan M. *The Protest Psychosis: How Schizophrenia Became a Black Disease*. Boston: Beacon Press, 2009.

Moore, Leonard Joseph. *Citizen Klansmen: The Ku Klux Klan in Indiana, 1921–1928*. Chapel Hill: University of North Carolina Press, 1992.

Morrison, Hazel. "Constructing Patient Stories: 'Dynamic' Case Notes and Clinical Encounters at Glasgow's Gartnavel Mental Hospital, 1921–32." *Medical History* 60, no. 1 (2016): 67–86.

Nielsen, Kim E. *A Disability History of the United States*. Boston: Beacon Press, 2012.

Nielsen, Kim E. *Money, Marriage, and Madness: The Life of Anna Ott*. Champaign: University of Illinois Press, 2020.

Nielsen, Kim E. "The Perils and Promises of Disability Biography." In Rembis, Kudlick, and Nielsen, *The Oxford Handbook of Disability History*, 21–40.

Nystrom, Kenneth C. "The Bioarchaeology of Structural Violence and Dissection in the 19th-Century United States." *American Anthropologist* 116, no. 4 (2014): 765–79.

Osgood, Robert L. "The Menace of the Feebleminded: George Bliss, Amos Butler, and the Indiana Committee on Mental Defectives." *Indiana Magazine of History* 97, no. 4 (2001): 253–77.

Parascandola, John. *Sex, Sin, and Science: A History of Syphilis in America*. Westport, CT: Praeger, 2008.

Parsons, Anne E. *From Asylum to Prison: Deinstitutionalization and the Rise of Mass Incarceration after 1945*. Chapel Hill: University of North Carolina Press, 2018.

Payne, Rodger M. "Adapting the Urban Parish: St. John the Evangelist Roman Catholic Church, Indianapolis, Indiana." *Anglican and Episcopal History* 64, no. 2 (1995): 255–59.

Peiss, Kathy. *Cheap Amusements: Working Women and Leisure in Turn-of-the-Century New York*. Philadelphia, PA: Temple University Press, 1987.

Pemberton, Stephen. "The Curious Case of the 'Professional Hemophiliac': Medicine, Disability, and the Contested Value of Normality in the United States, 1940–2010." In Burch and Rembis, *Disability Histories*, 237–57.

Poirier, Suzanne. *Chicago's War on Syphilis, 1937–1940: The Times, the "Trib," and the Clap Doctor*. Urbana: University of Illinois Press, 1995.

Porter, Roy. *A Social History of Madness: The World through the Eyes of the Insane*. London: Weidenfeld and Nicolson, 1987.

Probst, George Theodore. *The Germans in Indianapolis, 1840–1918*. Indianapolis: Indiana German Heritage Society, 1989.

Quétel, Claude. *History of Syphilis*. Baltimore, MD: Johns Hopkins University Press, 1990.

Reardon, Jenny. *The Postgenomic Condition: Ethics, Justice, and Knowledge after the Genome*. Chicago: University of Chicago Press, 2017.

Reaume, Geoffrey. "Mad People's History." *Radical History Review*, no. 94 (2006): 170–82.

Reaume, Geoffrey. *Remembrance of Patients Past: Patient Life at the Toronto Hospital for the Insane, 1890–1940*. New York: Oxford University Press, 2000.

Reilly, Philip R. *The Surgical Solution: A History of Involuntary Sterilization in the United States*. Baltimore, MD: Johns Hopkins University Press, 1991.

Rembis, Michael A. *Defining Deviance: Sex, Science, and Delinquent Girls, 1890–1960*. Urbana: University of Illinois Press, 2011.

Rembis, Michael A. "The New Asylums: Madness and Mass Incarceration in the Neoliberal Era." In Ben-Moshe, Chapman, and Carey, *Disability Incarcerated*, 139–59.

Rembis, Michael A. *Writing Mad Lives in the Age of the Asylum*. New York: Oxford University Press, forthcoming.

Rembis, Michael, Catherine Kudlick, and Kim E. Nielsen, eds. *The Oxford Handbook of Disability History*. New York: Oxford University Press, 2018.

Reverby, Susan M. *Examining Tuskegee: The Infamous Syphilis Study and Its Legacy*. Chapel Hill: University of North Carolina Press, 2009.

Reverby, Susan M. "Suffering and Resistance, Voice and Agency: Thoughts on History and the Tuskegee Syphilis Study." In *Precarious Prescriptions: Contested Histories of Race and Health in North America*, edited by Laurie B. Green, John McKiernan-González, and Martin Summers, 261–74. Minneapolis: University of Minnesota Press, 2014.

Richards, Penny L., and Susan Burch. "Documents, Ethics, and the Disability Historian." In Rembis, Kudlick, and Nielsen, *The Oxford Handbook of Disability History*, 161–76.

Roediger, David R. *Colored White: Transcending the Racial Past*. Berkeley: University of California Press, 2002.

Roediger, David R. *Working toward Whiteness: How America's Immigrants Became White; The Strange Journey from Ellis Island to the Suburbs*. New York: Basic Books, 2005.

Rosenberg, Charles E. *No Other Gods: On Science and American Social Thought*. Rev. ed. Baltimore, MD: Johns Hopkins University Press, 1997.

Rydell, Robert W., and Laura Burd Schiavo, eds. *Designing Tomorrow: America's World Fairs of the 1930s*. New Haven, CT: Yale University Press, 2010.

Sample, Bradford. "A Truly Midwestern City: Indianapolis on the Eve of the Great Depression." *Indiana Magazine of History* 97, no. 2 (June 2001): 129–47.

Sartin, Jeffrey S., and Harold O. Perry. "From Mercury to Malaria to Penicillin: The History of the Treatment of Syphilis at the Mayo Clinic—1916–1955." *Journal of the American Academy of Dermatology* 32, no. 2, part 1 (February 1995): 255–61.

Scull, Andrew. *Desperate Remedies: Psychiatry's Turbulent Quest to Cure Mental Illness*. Cambridge, MA: Belknap Press of Harvard University Press, 2022.

Scull, Andrew. *Madhouse: A Tragic Tale of Megalomania and Modern Medicine*. New Haven, CT: Yale University Press, 2005.

Sedgwick, Eve Kosofsky. *Touching Feeling: Affect, Pedagogy, Performativity*. Durham, NC: Duke University Press, 2003.

Sedgwick, Eve Kosofsky, and Adam Frank, eds. *Shame and Its Sisters: A Silvan Tomkins Reader*. Durham, NC: Duke University Press, 1995.

Shultz, Suzanne M. *Body Snatching: The Robbing of Graves for the Education of Physicians in Early Nineteenth Century America*. Jefferson, NC: McFarland, 1992.

Sleeper-Smith, Susan. "Resistance to Removal: The 'White Indian,' Frances Slocum." In Edmunds, *Enduring Nations*, 109–23.

Spandler, Helen, Jill Anderson, and Bob Sapey, eds. *Madness, Distress and the Politics of Disablement*. Bristol, UK: Policy Press, 2015.

Statistica. "Percentage of Housing Units with Telephones in the United States from 1920 to 2008." Published September 30, 2010. https://www.statista.com/statistics/189959/.

StatsIndiana. "Indiana City/Town Census Counts, 1900–2010." Accessed February 14, 2024. http://www.stats.indiana.edu/population/PopTotals/historic_counts_cities.asp.

Stearns, Peter N. *Shame: A Brief History*. Urbana: University of Illinois Press, 2017.

Stern, Alexandra Minna. *Eugenic Nation: Faults and Frontiers of Better Breeding in Modern America*. 2nd ed. Oakland: University of California Press, 2016.

Stern, Alexandra Minna. "From Legislation to Lived Experience: Eugenic Sterilization in California and Indiana 1907–1979." In Lombardo, *A Century of Eugenics in America*, 95–116.

Stern, Alexandra Minna. "'We Cannot Make a Silk Purse Out of a Sow's Ear': Eugenics in the Hoosier Heartland." *Indiana Magazine of History* 103, no. 1 (March 2007): 3–38.

Stern, Scott W. *The Trials of Nina McCall: Sex, Surveillance, and the Decades-Long Government Plan to Imprison "Promiscuous" Women*. Boston: Beacon Press, 2018.

Summers, Martin. "'Suitable Care of the African When Afflicted with Insanity': Race, Madness, and Social Order in Comparative Perspective." *Bulletin of the History of Medicine* 84, no. 1 (2010): 58–91.

Sussman, Robert Wald. *The Myth of Race: The Troubling Persistence of an Unscientific Idea*. Cambridge, MA: Harvard University Press, 2014.

Tomes, Nancy. *Remaking the American Patient: How Madison Avenue and Modern Medicine Turned Patients into Consumers*. Chapel Hill: University of North Carolina Press, 2016.

Trouillot, Michel-Rolph. *Silencing the Past: Power and the Production of History*. Boston: Beacon Press, 1995.

Tsay, Cynthia J. "Julius Wagner-Jauregg and the Legacy of Malarial Therapy for the Treatment of General Paresis of the Insane." *Yale Journal of Biology and Medicine* 86, no. 2 (2013): 245–54.

Tuggle, Lindsey. *The Afterlives of Specimens: Science, Mourning, and Whitman's Civil War*. Iowa City: University of Iowa Press, 2017.

Wailoo, Keith. *Dying in the City of the Blues: Sickle Cell Anemia and the Politics of Race and Health*. Chapel Hill: University of North Carolina Press, 2001.

Washington, Harriet A. *Medical Apartheid: The Dark History of Medical Experimentation on Black Americans from Colonial Times to the Present*. New York: Anchor Books, 2006.

Watson, Nick, Alan Roulstone, and Carol Thomas, eds. *Routledge Handbook of Disability Studies*. 2nd ed. New York: Routledge, 2020.

Whitaker, Robert. *Mad in America: Bad Science, Bed Medicine, and the Enduring Mistreatment of the Mentally Ill*. Cambridge, MA: Perseus, 2002.

Whitrow, Magda. *Julius Wagner-Jauregg (1857–1940)*. London: Smith-Gordon, 1993.

Whitrow, Magda. "Wagner-Jauregg and Fever Therapy." *Medical History* 34, no. 3 (1990): 294–310.

World Health Organization. "Malaria." Fact sheet. Updated March 29, 2023. https://www.who.int/news-room/fact-sheets/detail/malaria.

Yudell, Michael. *Race Unmasked: Biology and Race in the Twentieth Century*. New York: Columbia University Press, 2014.

Zwicker, Katherine. "Experimenting with Radium Therapy: In the Laboratory and the Clinic." In Dyck and Stewart, *The Uses of Humans in Experiment*, 194–214.

Index

Note: Page numbers in *italics* denotes figures.

ableism, 4, 9–10, 64–66, 96–98, 105, 120
Adams, Heather Brook, 126n19, 135n88
Agnew, Anna, 34, 36
Allison, Anthony C., 147n44
American Medical Association, 48, 110
American Social Hygiene Association (ASHA), 30–31
anatomy laws, 105, 107–10
Anopheles mosquitos, 50, 138n54
Ariès, Philippe, 105, 118, 149n11
arsenicals, 1, 33, 42–43, 50, 54–55, 77
Asylum of Lower Austria (Vienna), 43
autopsy/dissection: Americans' views of, 17, 106–9, 115–18; Bruetsch's role in, 7, 10, 52–53, 77–78, 80–81, 91, 117–18; in CSH malaria research, 14, 52–53, 77, 104, 106, 109–16; disambiguated, 111–13; family consent/refusal for, 64, 74–75, 103, 105–6, 109, 112–14, 116–17, 141n34; marginalized/unclaimed bodies and, 107–9, 111–14, 117; medical education's use of, 107–13, *111*, 117–18, 149n10;

specific instances of, 52–53, 71, 73, 77, 100, 112–13, 117

Bahr, Max: on autopsy, 12, 104–6, 109, 112–14, 116; on CSH workings/legacy, 48–49, 53–54, 57, 65–67, 70–72; cure sought by, 40, 43–44, 57, 59–60, 96–97; on eugenics/public health reform, 12, 29–30, 96–97, 101; life/work of, 38–41, *39*, 44–45, 122; on malaria therapy treatment, 17, 37, 48–49, 51–52, 54, 76–77, 80, 143n86; on neurosyphilis rates, 29–30, 40, 125n4, 134n87; patient consent/advocacy and, 64, 74–75, 105–6, 114; racial/gendered biases of, 84, 88–90, 92–93
Bell, Joseph E., 20–22, 28
Ben-Moshe, Liat, 67, 128n42
biological determinism, 85–86, 89–91, 93
Birzer, Bradley J., 137n39
Blackness/Black communities, 46–47, 85–91, 107–8, 112–13
Black syphilis patients: at CSH, 84–93; in Tuskegee, 5, 11, 85–86, 89–93, 120
bodily autonomy, 64, 73–75, 98–102, 107–10
body snatching, 107–8

Index

Bonner, Thomas Neville, 136n16
Boston Psychopathic Hospital, 67
Boyd, Mark, 5, 89, 91
Braslow, Joel, 5, 68, 135n3
Bruetsch, Walter L.: CSH's treatment protocol and, 50–56, 76–79, 92; cure sought by, 10, 40, 44, 56–57, 59–60, 96–97; dissection by, 7–8, 10, 104, 110, 113; German tour of (1930–31), 37–38, 53, 57, 116–17; life/work of, 13–14, 38, 40–42, *41*, 44–46, 121–22; Mabel Smith and, 36, 37–38, 119; medical conclusions of, 52–54, 76, 79–81, 84, 88–89; patient consent/advocacy and, 64–66, 74; postmortem notes of, 52–53, 77–78, 80–81, 91, 113–16; racial/gendered biases of, 84, 88–93, 99–100, 122; reputation of, 9–10, 12–13, 48–49, 53–55, 66–67, 122
Buck v. Bell, 100
Bunker, Henry A., Jr., 138n60, 139n68
Burch, Susan, 128n44

cadaver usage, 107–13, 117–18, 149n10
Cahn, Susan K., 128n40
carceral medicine: conceptualized, 67; erasure/silencing of patient stories in, 9–10, 18–20, 60, 105, 118; gender constructions reinforced by, 83–84, 93–98; pregnancy/sterilization and, 98–102; racial constructions reinforced by, 83–86, 89–93; resisted by patients/families, 72–75; terror/distress/danger of, 9–10, 67–73, 81
Cardozo, Benjamin, 64
Carey, Allison C., 128n42
Catholicism, 4–5, 7, 20, 22–25, 116–17, 123–24
Central State Hospital for the Insane (CSH): Bahr and Bruetsch's shaping of, 38–41, 44–45, 121–22; Black patients at, 84–93; carceral medicine at, 9–10, 67–73; as educational hub, 51, 66–67, 109–12, *111*, 117–18; grounds/campus of, 1, 66, *78*, *94*, 105, 124; incomplete/inaccurate records of, 18, 73–74, 105, 114–15, 141n34; as leader in experimental malaria therapy, 7–9, 37–38, 48–49, 51, 53–55, 57, 79; malaria therapy protocol at, 17–18, 50–56, 76–79, 136n20; marginalized patients at, 83–84, 111–13, 117, 122–23; pathology at, 7, 38, 57, *78*, 104–6, 109–16, *111*; patient consent practices at, 64–66, 74, 99–101, 105–6, 112–14; staff turnover/overcrowding at, 33, 62, 69–73; success/efficacy rate, 2, 51, 59–60, 79, 81, 97–98; women patients at, 33–35, 66, 93–101, *94*. See also Bahr, Max; Bruetsch, Walter L.
—Patient experiences: death, 52–53, 56, 71–73, 77–78, 91, 101, 114–16; disregarded by physicians, 51, 77–78, 80, 95–96, 99, 120, 122–23; distress/embarrassment/suffering, 68–69, 73, 79–81, 95–96; inconsistent malaria therapy application, 76–79, 89–91, 115; neurosyphilis symptoms, 11, 42–43, 59–63; pregnancy/sterilization, 98–102; rehabilitation/employment and, 96–98, 120; resistance efforts and, 72–75; segregated housing, 93–94, 145n22
Chain, Ernst, 55
Chapman, Chris, 128n42
Charité Hospital (Berlin), 39
Christian Science, 74
City Hospital (Indianapolis), *32*; funding/administration of, 31–33, 46; Mabel Smith at, 1, 17, 31, 33, 37; other patients at, 51, 61, 63, 81, 87–88, 109
Civil War, 85, 106–7
Clarke, Walter, 31
Commission on Training Camp Activities (CTCA), 29, 31
Committee on Research in Syphilis, 50, 67
consent: informed, 10, 60, 64; presence/absence of, 64–66, 74, 99–101, 105–6, 109, 112–14

consumer culture, 22–23, 26–28
Cooperative Clinical Group Study, 50, 67
Cormack, James, 24
Cotton, Henry, 136n17
Council of Social Agencies, 27
county jails, 30, 33, 61–62
Crenner, Christopher, 144n10
cure, 2, 38, 42–44, 56–57, 81–82, 96–98, 114, 120

Dalton, Katherine (Killila), 20, 23, 60, 116, 123–24
Dalton, Michael, 20–23, 60, 116, 123–24
Davis, Gayle, 79, 125n2
death: cadaver/autopsy material, 107–18, 149n10; shifting perceptions of, 104–9, 115–18, 151n56; silenced/erased, 103–5, 118. See also autopsy/dissection
defectiveness, 27, 29–30, 34, 84
degeneracy, 9, 17, 21, 27–29, 76, 84–85, 95, 97, 120
de-lineating, 4–5, 13, 104, 120
D'Emilio, John, 130n24, 131n31
Democratic Party politics, 20–23
Demos, John, 126n15
deviance, 20, 27–28, 34, 134n86
diathermy, 91
Dibble, Eugene H., Jr., 5, 89–92
disability: acquired, 5, 18, 35, 61–62, 65–66, 77, 83; diagnostic regimes of, 134n86; Down syndrome, 4–5; family shame/silence and, 3–5, 14, 18, 103–4, 118; identity reduced to, 69; transgressive sexuality as, 27, 29
dissection. See autopsy/dissection
Dix, Dorothea, 33
domesticity, 19, 23, 84, 94–95, 97
Donaldson, Elizabeth J., 8
Dorr, Gregory M., 144n3
Dyck, Erika, 128n35, 128n43, 144n4

Edenharter, George F., 40
Edmunds, R. David, 137n37
Ehrlich, Paul, 42
Eldridge, Watson W., 139n68

electroconvulsive treatment, 35
Eugenics Record Office, 30
eugenic thinking: Catholicism's intersection with, 131n29; on degeneracy, 27–29; disempowerment of "unfit," 3, 11–12, 21–22, 30, 35, 76, 84, 98, 101, 120; financial arguments for, 29–30, 41, 96–97; gendered expectations and, 34–35, 84, 93–98; hereditarianism, 76, 84, 102, 120; marriage laws and, 12, 100–101; medical racism and, 14, 84–86, 120–21; public health goals of, 11–12, 27–30; sterilization, 98–102; Wagner-Jauregg's embrace of, 44

Faust, Drew Gilpin, 149n11, 149n13
feeblemindedness, 27, 76, 101, 128n142, 132n47
feminist disability studies: author's framework of, 2–3, 6–10, 12–15, 19–20, 60–61, 119, 124; re-lineating and, 4–5, 13, 120, 124
fever therapy, 2, 43
Fields, Barbara J., 92–93, 144n6, 145n24
Fields, Karen E., 92–93, 144n6, 145n24
Fink, Jennifer Natalya, 4–5
Fleming, Alexander, 55
Florey, Howard, 55
Fort Wayne State School, 101
Foster, Eugene, 31
Fox, Renée C., 148n63
Freedman, Estelle B., 130n24, 131n31

Galen, 43
Gallagher-Cohoon, Erin, 147n46
Gambino, Matthew, 5, 141n28, 147n43
Geller, Jeffrey L., 127n27, 134n85
gender norms/ideology: domesticity, 19, 23, 84, 94–95, 97; interwar shifts in, 26–28, 34–35, 93, 123; pregnancy/childbirth, 18, 22–25, 98–102, 123, 147n46; productive labor and, 84, 93–94, 96–98, 102, 120. See also transgressive sexuality; women syphilis patients

general paralysis of the insane. *See* neurosyphilis
German Psychiatric Association, 53
Glass, James, 131n27
Gordon, Linda, 145n19
Government Emergency Hospital (Washington, DC), 39
grave robbing, 107–8
Great Depression, 59
Great Migration, 46–47
Grob, Gerald, 128n48, 135n9

Halpern, Sydney A., 141n31
Harris, Maxine, 127n27, 134n85
Harrison, John Scott, 108
Harrison, William Henry, 108
Helgeson, Jeffrey, 137n44
hereditarianism, 76, 84, 102, 120
HIPAA, 129n58
Hippocrates, 43
Holy Cross and Saint Joseph Cemetery, 123–24
Hull-House, 32
Humphrey, David C., 150n19
Humphreys, Margaret, 5, 89, 139n62
hysteria, 96

Imada, Adria L., 67
incarceration. *See* carceral medicine
Indiana: anatomy laws, 105, 107–10; eugenics policy/laws, 12, 29–30, 98, 100–102; Indigenous peoples of, 45, 47; moral panic in, 26–29
Indiana Committee on Mental Defectives, 30
Indiana Medical History Museum, 7, 9, 78, 149n7
Indianapolis: anti-syphilis efforts, 30–33; city politics of, 20–22, 28, 31, 46; history/demographics of, 20, 44–48, 86–88; leisure activities in, 22–23, 27–28; Mabel Smith's life/community in, 7, 20–25, 116, 123–24. *See also individual hospitals/organizations*
Indianapolis Board of Health, 31
Indianapolis Foundation, 27–28, 30–33, 87–88, 130n19, 145n17

Indiana State Anatomical Board, 108
Indiana State Archives, 4, 8
Indiana University School of Medicine, 110, 112
Indigenous peoples, 45, 47
informed consent. *See* consent
insanity/madness: biological causes recognized, 11, 29–30, 35, 39–42; Black vs. white, 86, 89; immorality viewed as cause of, 11, 29–30, 42, 95; inability to consent and, 64–66, 74, 99–101; label of, 34, 128n35; women's experiences of, 8–9, 34–35, 96, 124
institutionalization: as dehumanizing/disabling, 68–69, 83, 107–16; shame of, 103–4; women's, 27, 29, 33–35, 66, 93–100, 94. *See also* carceral medicine
insulin shock treatment, 35
interwar era: institutionalizations during, 34–35, 93; laboratory science during, 29, 39–42, 49, 65, 116; moral panic, 26–29, 34; nativism/racism, 25–26, 44, 46–47; social reformers of, 11–12, 27–30, 101

Jackson, Frederick, 31
Jefferson, Thomas, 144n6
John A. Andrew Memorial Hospital (Tuskegee), 85–86, 90–91
Johns Hopkins Medical School, 121
Johnson, Bascom, 31
Journal of Nervous and Mental Disease, 52
Journal of the American Medical Association, 56

Keifetz, Lorie, 4
Kirby, George H., 138n60, 139n68
Kobrowski, Nicole R., 145n22, 149n7, 151n34
Kudlick, Catherine, 125n7
Ku Klux Klan, 87–88, 132n44

Laderman, Gary, 149n6, 150n28
leisure time, 22–23, 26–28

Leon, Sharon M., 131n29
Lies, Eugene T., 27–28
Lincoln, Abraham, 149n13
Lombardo, Paul A., 144n3
Lynd, Robert and Helen, 26, 28

madness. *See* insanity/madness
mad studies, 6
malaria: community spread of, 47–48, 50–51; imagined Black immunity to, 89–91, 147n44; quartan/tertiary, 89–91, 136n28
malaria therapy treatment: vs. alternative treatments/nontreatment, 55–57, 67, 77–78, 89–92, 120–21; autopsy's role in, 104, 106, 109–16; CSH protocol for, 17–18, 50–56, 76–79, 136n20; CSH's leading role in, 7–9, 37–38, 44–45, 48–49, 51, 53–54, 66–67, 79; ethical considerations of, 43–44, 48, 57, 64–66, 99–100, 122; gender and, 84, 93–100; historical context of, 5, 10–12; Mabel Smith's experience with, 18, 35–36; medical racism and, 84, 86–93, 102, 120–21; national variations in, 49–50, 54; power inequalities and, 2–3, 6–7, 9–10, 13–14, 60, 64–66, 69, 74–75, 81, 120–21; risks to patient/society, 48, 50–51, 77–81, 91, 99–100, 115, 122; success/efficacy rates of, 2, 51, 59–60, 79, 81, 97–98; Wagner-Jauregg's research into, 2, 43–44, 50
Malaria Treatment of General Paralysis, The, 53
malaria tropica, 43
male syphilis patients, 8, 93–96
Manhattan State Hospital (New York), 49–50
marriage blood test law, 12, 100–101
Mayo Clinic, 67, 139n68
Medical College of Georgia, 112–13
medical experimentation: autopsy as key to, 104, 106; bodies as data/specimens, 14–15, 38, 40, 53, 60, 65, 68–69, 84–86, 88, 91–93, 109–16;

bodies as instruments, 128n43; clinical/research overlap, 49–50, 54, 60, 65–66, 77–78, 91–92, 99, 116, 122; ethical considerations of, 43–44, 48, 57, 64–66, 85, 90–91, 99–100, 122; individual researcher's centrality to, 49–50, 122, 136n17; power inequalities and, 60, 64–66, 81, 106–8; "success" despite patient deaths, 52–53, 66–67, 77–79. *See also* malaria therapy treatment; Tuskegee syphilis study
medical incarceration. *See* carceral medicine
medical/scientific racism: after death, 107–8, 112–13; Bruetsch's research and, 14, 84, 88–93; history of, 85–86; hospital segregation, 47, 87–88
Methodist Hospital (Indianapolis), 151n34
Metzl, Jonathan M., 145n14, 147n62
Miami Tribe, 45
Middletown (Lynd and Lynd), 26, 28
Miller, Anne, 55–56
moral panic, 26–29, 34. *See also* shame; transgressive sexuality
Morris, Dr., 77
Morrison, Hazel, 127n33, 144n1
mosquitos, 48, 50
Muscatatuck State School, 101

National Research Council, 55, 67, 92, 121
Nazism, 44
Neosalvarsan, 33, 136n20
neurosyphilis: cerebral hemorrhage, 24, 102; "cure" sought for, 38, 42–44, 56, 81–82, 96–98; emaciation, 59–60; glossed, 1, 17; hallucinations/delusions of grandiosity, 11, 42, 61–63, 88; pregnancy and, 99–100; racial disparities, 86, 89; remissions/relapses, 51, 81, 97–98, 136n31, 139nn67–68; violent outbursts/actions, 62–63, 68–69, 76. *See also* malaria therapy treatment; shame; syphilis

New York State Psychiatric Institute, 51
Nielsen, Kim E., 127n28, 127nn30–31
Nobel Prize, 43–44
normalcy, 2–3, 6, 13, 18, 27, 92, 97–99, 101–2, 113

Ohio Medical College, 108
O'Leary, Paul A., 139n68

Paget's disease, 112–13
pain, theorized, 68, 80, 120, 123
paresis. *See* neurosyphilis
Parran, Thomas, 11, 144n10
Parsons, Anne E., 145n22, 147n46
penicillin, 55–57, 67, 85, 90, 92, 121
physician "beneficence," 8, 65–66, 81, 122
physician-patient relationship, 57, 63, 68–69, 135n3
Plasmodium falciparum, 91
Plasmodium vivax, 89
Poirier, Suzanne, 136n25, 140n8
pregnancy/childbirth, 18, 22–25, 98–102, 123, 147n46
Prenatti, Francis, 37, 103
progress (medical/scientific), 38, 41, 59–60, 90, 101, 120–22, 148n63
Progressive Era, 9–11, 21–23, 26, 28, 46, 48
promiscuity. *See* transgressive sexuality
prostitution, 23, 26, 29, 31
psychiatry/psychiatrists: autopsy material used for, 110, 112; on Black vs. white madness, 86, 89; Germany at vanguard of, 2, 38–44, 53; pathologizing of women by, 8, 34, 124; perceptions of insanity, 11, 29–30, 35, 39–42. *See also* carceral medicine
public health/social reformers, 11–12, 27–30, 46, 101

quartan malaria, 91, 136n28
quinine, 18, 43, 50–51, 76, 80

racecraft, 92–93
racism, 25–26, 44, 46–47, 86–88. *See also* medical/scientific racism
radium cancer therapy, 65
Reardon, Jenny, 152n57
Reaume, Geoffrey, 127n27, 127n33
re-lineating, 4–5, 13, 120, 124
Rembis, Michael, 9, 27, 127n27, 132n47, 134n83
reproductive lives, 18, 22–25, 98–102, 123, 147n46
resurrectionists, 107–8
Reverby, Susan M., 5, 90, 140n7
Robert W. Long Hospital (Indianapolis), 100
Rockefeller Foundation, 55

Saint Elizabeths Hospital (Washington, DC), 5, 39, 49–50, 64, 86, 138n56, 147n43
Saint Vincent Hospital (Indianapolis), 47, 145n17
Salvarsan (arsphenamine), 1, 33, 42–43, 50, 54, 77
schizophrenia, 35, 78
scientific racism. *See* medical/scientific racism
Scull, Andrew, 136n31, 136nn16–17
Sedgwick, Eve Kosofsky, 126n14
segregation (racial/sex), 47, 87–88, 93–94
Seven Steeples, *66, 93, 94*
shame: ableism's role in shaping, 4, 9–10, 105; conceptualized, 3, 23, 127n23; of death, 103–5, 118, 123; denial/forgetting and, 130n9; families' experience of, 62–63, 104; family erasure, 3–5, 12, 14, 18, 20, 23–25, 103–4, 118, 119–20, 123–24; gendered, 1–2, 8, 13, 18, 26–29, 34–35, 84, 94–96; historical/medical erasure and, 8, 18–19, 23, 35, 103–5, 118, 119–20, 124, 131n34; medical attendants' experience of, 70–71; stigma of syphilis and, 1–2, 8, 11–12, 18, 29–31, 35, 83, 103–4; of transgressive sexuality, 2, 5, 18, 23, 34–35

Shultz, Suzanne M., 151n56
sickle cell anemia, 93, 145n15
Sleeper-Smith, Susan, 137n40
Smith, Arthur, 1, 18, 24–25, 33, 60, 116
Smith, Mabel (Katherine Mabel Dalton Ward Smith): author's relation to, 3–4, 6–7, 14, 19, 120, 125n3; book's ethical project and, 12–14, 83, 120, 124; Bruetsch and, 36, 37–38, 119; at City Hospital, 1, 17, 31, 33, 37; CSH admission/treatment of, 1, 4, 17–18, 34–36, 59–61; decline/death of, 37–38, 57, 103, 116–17, *117*, 119, 121, 123; family/historical silence, 3–5, 7–8, 14, 18, 20, 23–25, 103–4, 119–20, 123–24; life of, 5, 7, 13, *19*, 20–25, 98, 101–2; transgressive sexual history of, 18, 22–25, 35, 123
staphylococcal bacteria, 51
Stearns, Peter N., 3, 123, 126n19, 130n9, 132n44
sterilization, 98–102
Stern, Alexandra Minna, 133n55
Stewart, Larry, 128n43
St. John the Evangelist Catholic Church, 7, 20, 23–25, 47, 123–24
Stockton, Sarah, 34
Stovarsol, 54–55, 136n20
streptococcus, 43
Swazey, Judith P., 148n63
syphilis: arsenicals/early-stage treatments, 1, 11, 33, 42–43, 50, 54–55, 77; congenital/familial, 24, 75–76, 101–2; federal/local efforts against, 28–33, 41; German research into, 42–44; institutionalization rates and, 1, 29–30, 35, 40; racial disparities, 86, 89; shame of, 1–2, 8, 11–12, 18, 29–31, 35, 83, 103–4; Wassermann diagnostic test, 42, 73, 88, 95, 115, 128n47. *See also* neurosyphilis; venereal disease
syphilis spirochete, 42, 52, 54, 122, 128n47

tertian malaria, 89–91
Tidwell, Dr., 17, 33
Tomkins, Silvan, 123, 127n23, 134n84
transgressive sexuality: masturbation, 95; premarital/extramarital sex, 18, 22–23, 25, 35, 99, 123, 126n20; promiscuity, 2, 5, 26–29, 94–96; shame of, 2, 5, 18, 23, 34–35
Trenton State Hospital, 136n17
Tsay, Cynthia J., 136n27, 137n33
tuberculin, 43
Tuggle, Lindsey, 149n13
Turner, Thomas B., 121
Tuskegee syphilis study, 5, 11, 85–86, 89–93, 120
typhoid fever, 77–78

ultraviolet radiation, 54–55
US Public Health Service, 11, 85, 147n46
US Supreme Court, 100

Van Meter, F. J., 138n56
Vehling, Fred W., 109
venereal disease: medical racism and, 85–87; public health campaigns and, 11, 30–32; shame/stigma of, 26–29, 34–35, 84, 94–96, 101–2, 103–4. *See also* neurosyphilis; syphilis
Veterans Hospital (Tuskegee), 5, 90–92
vice, 21–23, 26, 28, 30

Wagner-Jauregg, Julius, 2, 7, 40, 42–44, 50
Wailoo, Keith, 145n15, 147n44
Walsh, William H., 145n17
Ward, Charles Irvin (Jack Poole), 22–24, 102, 123
Washington, Harriet A., 112, 150n16
Wassermann, August von, 42
Wassermann test, 1, 17, 42, 73, 88, 95, 115
whiteness/white communities, 25, 44–48, 83, 85–88, 90

Whitman, Walt, 149n13
Whitrow, Magda, 136n28
Wilborn, Bessie, 112–13
women physicians, 34
women syphilis patients: in CSH's Seven Steeples, 66, 93, 94; gendered shame and, 2, 8, 13, 18, 29, 35; madness experienced by, 8–9; patient intake forms and, 93–96; pregnancy/sterilization of, 98–102; vectors of infection and, 28–29, 101–2. *See also* gender norms/ideology; transgressive sexuality

working class, 4–5, 18, 22–23, 83

World War I, 11, 28–29, 31, 39–40, 43, 46, 89, 101

World War II, 11, 56

Zwicker, Katherine, 65

CHRISTIN L. HANCOCK is a professor of history and gender, women, and sexuality studies at the University of Portland and associate dean for curriculum in the College of Arts and Sciences.

The University of Illinois Press
is a founding member of the
Association of University Presses.

———————————————

Composed in 10.5/13.5 Mercury Text G2
with Avenir LT Std display
by Kirsten Dennison
at the University of Illinois Press

University of Illinois Press
1325 South Oak Street
Champaign, IL 61820-6903
www.press.uillinois.edu